Brain Imaging

Brain Imaging

What It Can (and Cannot) Tell Us About Consciousness

Robert G. Shulman

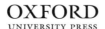
OXFORD
UNIVERSITY PRESS

OXFORD
UNIVERSITY PRESS

Oxford University Press is a department of the University of Oxford.
It furthers the University's objective of excellence in research, scholarship,
and education by publishing worldwide.

Oxford   New York
Auckland   Cape Town   Dar es Salaam   Hong Kong   Karachi
Kuala Lumpur   Madrid   Melbourne   Mexico City   Nairobi
New Delhi   Shanghai   Taipei   Toronto

With offices in
Argentina   Austria   Brazil   Chile   Czech Republic   France   Greece
Guatemala   Hungary   Italy   Japan   Poland   Portugal   Singapore
South Korea   Switzerland   Thailand   Turkey   Ukraine   Vietnam

Oxford is a registered trademark of Oxford University Press in the UK and certain other
countries.

Published in the United States of America by
Oxford University Press
198 Madison Avenue, New York, NY 10016

© Oxford University Press 2013

Library of Congress Cataloging-in-Publication Data
Shulman, R. G. (Robert Gerson)
Brain imaging : what it can (and cannot) tell us about consciousness / Robert G. Shulman.
   pages cm
Includes bibliographical references and index.
ISBN 978–0–19–983872–1
1. Brain—Imaging.   2. Neurosciences.   I. Title.
QP376.6.S58 2013
612.8′2—dc23
2012046107

9 8 7 6 5 4 3
Printed in the United States of America
on acid-free paper

CONTENTS

Introduction

———

The progress of noninvasive nuclear magnetic resonance (NMR) methods over the past 30 years has been a stunning story of our growing ability to look into the complexities of brain chemistry and physics. As someone who has seen magnetic resonance progress from a crude tool that could measure water in the 1950s and simple biomolecules in the 1960s to the powerful lens it offers today for the study of *in vivo* brain activities and metabolism, I can testify to the astonishing progress that we have made. In this time, NMR methods have become tools for diagnosis in clinical medicine, for following metabolism *in vivo*, and for measuring changes in brain activity during stimulation. This multidirectional expansion of our ability to analyze physical and chemical activities within living beings has moved scientific inquiry to the inner workings of the living human—to study the force of muscle, the chemistry of liver, the malfunctions of diseases—and, recently, to that most fascinating of all activities, the function of the human brain. In contrast to the muscle, liver, heart, and kidney, all of which can be excised from the body and maintained in a living state on the bench top, the brain must be studied in the living person. The possibilities of noninvasive studies of brain activity *in vivo* have created a wave of excitement in neuroscience, and rightfully so.

NMR, the method of choice for *in vivo* studies, has been central in my entire career. The early homemade electronic equipment, interfaced with permanent magnets whose steel faces we hand-polished with sandpaper, has been replaced by superconducting magnets and by spectrometers of unimagined sensitivity, controlled by computers of equally undreamt-of ability. Improvements in equipment for data acquisition were much needed because the NMR signal is very weak compared to thermal noise. However, the very weakness of the signal has been responsible for the value of the method. The radio waves that readily penetrate matter such as air, buildings, or tissue are very weak compared to other electromagnetic waves like visible light, ultraviolet, and x-rays, and therefore they do not disturb the atoms and molecules surrounding the nuclei that are being detected.

THREE FORMS OF NMR

NMR is a form of spectroscopy in which the nuclei in a material, placed in a magnetic field, exchange energy with radiofrequency electromagnetic waves. Invented by physicists as a method for studying nuclear properties, it soon became of wide value in chemistry, condensed-matter physics, geology, and biochemistry, and more recently it has become a fundamental method for studying the properties of tissue *in vivo*. How we can (and might) frame our experiments utilizing noninvasive NMR studies of humans and animals *in vivo*, particularly of their otherwise inaccessible brains, is the subject of this book. The applications of NMR to noninvasive studies of humans and animals *in vivo* are served by a rich variety of methods. The first NMR method recognized to be valuable in human studies was magnetic resonance imaging (MRI), which provided a three-dimensional image of H_2O molecules *in vivo*. Within a decade of its demonstration in principle in test tubes by Paul Lauterbur,[1] international meetings were organized by neurologists, cardiologists, neuroscientists, and the rag-tail group of NMR specialists and computer scientists who had been developing MRI methods and interpretations. MRI was extended in the early 1990s to functional MRI (fMRI), which located changes in brain activity in response to stimulations of the person.[2,3] These experiments were based upon Seiji Ogawa's proposal[4] that changes in the degree of oxygenation of hemoglobin could be detected in MRI maps. Since these signals came from coupled changes in cerebral blood flow and oxygen consumption, they contained information about metabolic responses to stimulation. fMRI responses of the human visual cortex to sensory stimuli reproducing and extending previous invasive animal studies, mainly of cats and nonhuman primates, and noninvasive human studies by positron emission tomography (PET)[5] created a widespread excitement about the possible uses of fMRI for the study of more complex responses of the human brain. The quantitative understanding of fundamental metabolic pathways reached by these *in vivo* experiments has built upon and gone far beyond the knowledge that could be found in the biochemistry textbooks from studies of extracts. *In vivo* metabolism was studied directly by magnetic resonance spectroscopy (MRS), which followed the flow of labeled ^{13}C compound through metabolic pools.[6]

BRAIN ENERGY AND WORK

My interest in cerebral metabolism were formed by early MRS studies of glucose metabolism in yeast and muscle in the 1970s at Bell Telephone Laboratories, where, with an enthusiastic group of young colleagues (Seiji Ogawa, Kamil Ugurbil, Gil

Navon, Tetsue Yamane, Jan den Hollander, and others), we established methods for following glucose metabolism in the primary energy-producing pathways. It took 20 years until larger magnets, better computers, improved spectroscopic techniques, and the advances made by several young collaborators at Yale, particularly Douglas Rothman and Kevin Behar, produced well-resolved, high-quality spectra of metabolites in the human brain. Once such spectra were available, the metabolic pathways of the brain, more complex than yeast or skeletal muscle but built upon the same basic reactions of glucose oxidation, provided information about the specifically cerebral activities of neuronal firing. By the early 1990s, brain spectra measuring the flow of the ^{13}C label from glucose to glutamate could be directly interpreted to give the flux into the Krebs cycle and the cerebral metabolic rate of glucose oxidation.

More improvements in spectral acquisition measured the flow from glutamate to glutamine, a flux that provided the rate of neuronal firing. Most neuronal firing in the human brain releases the neurotransmitter glutamate, which is recognized by the postsynaptic neuron. The glutamate is then picked up by nearby glial cells, which convert it to glutamine and eventually recycle it to the presynaptic neurons. The flux of neurotransmitter glutamate to glutamine, obtained from these spectra, determined the rates of neuronal firing. Each experiment measured both the rate of energy production by the oxidation of glucose and the rate of work done by neurotransmitter cycling.[7] Energy and work in the brain provided an understanding similar to that obtained by studying the same parameters in cardiac and skeletal muscle: namely, how the brain consumes nutrients, how brain activity affects the rates of energy consumed and fuel delivery, and how increased energy demands are handled during stimulation. The metabolic ^{13}C measurements, in conjunction with PET measurements and the existing lore of neurophysiology, moved brain studies into thermodynamics, and the brain became an organ whose work made chemical and physical sense. It provided opportunities for physical scientists to build a bottom-up understanding of brain functions from measurements of the energy consumed and the work of neuronal firing.

The following chapters describe how neurophysiology, attending to the chemical and physical brain properties described by imaging experiments, provides reliable physical understanding of mechanisms that support tentative proposals about relations between brain energetics and human behavior.

BUILDING UPON BEHAVIORISM

By confining attention to brain processes that are necessary for the person to perform observed behaviors, and by not studying mental processes postulated to relate brain activities to the observed behavior, my approach has some similarities with the once-popular school of psychology called Behaviorism. While there are similarities in our dependence upon observable behavior, our methods differ significantly from this older psychology as well as from the more recent cognitive psychology. J. B. Watson's definitive summary[8] showed the reliable role of behavior in science. Watson started with the clear statement, "Behavior can be observed like the phenomena of all other natural sciences." When controlled experiments established the connection between stimulus and response, then, Watson continued, the behaviorist's psychological questions have been answered. Not being able to observe in these investigations any mental processes, like "consciousness, sensation, perception, imagery or will," behaviorists, Watson writes, "reached the conclusion that all such terms can be dropped out of the description of man's activity." He continued: "the neurologists and physical chemists have problems to solve about the neuronal connections and in determining the physical and chemical work done in the reaction." However, he adds, those are not the concern of psychology, which he felt could be best pursued as the study of behavior. Watson does not conclude that mental processes do not exist, or that the brain played no role in supporting them— quite the contrary: he assumed they did but did not think that psychology had the tools to study them. That was close to a century ago. In the 1970s cognitive psychology started to fill the gap between stimulus and response by proposing both the nature of these mental processes and the brain mechanism for dealing with them from the perspective of computers, information theory, and linguistics. I share Watson's enthusiasm about the reliable explanatory powers of observable behavior and, as a Pragmatist, share his skepticism about the value of assuming mental processes. As a modern representative of the "neurologists" and physical chemists to whom he defers, I believe that physical scientists should study mechanisms of brain activity supporting a person's behavior rather than invoking mental processes responsible for that behavior. Freed from the need to answer questions that have been the responsibility of psychology, I have turned to neurophysiological studies of brain energy and work for insights into the neuronal support for behavioral activities.

THE NEED FOR PHILOSOPHY

Scientific directions exploring how brain experiments can be related to behavior and mental activity are intricately interdependent with philosophical issues that influence the choice of questions addressed and the methods used for their study. A scientist involved in neuroimaging studies can choose between many well-developed philosophical positions on issues of mind. Because mental activities have been so thoroughly integrated into social sciences, religion, and our culture, an individual cannot avoid taking a position on brain contributions to mental processes, so that the choice is not whether or not we follow a philosophical position but rather whether we do so knowingly or unthinkingly.

In a recent Tanner Lecture at Yale, Rebecca Goldstein, a novelist and philosopher, addressed the apparent differences between writing fiction, generally recognized as a creative personal activity, and the commitment to a philosophy, often pictured as an impersonal, rational, logical choice. The reality, she claimed, was quite different in that there was no subject more personal, more dependent upon individual preferences, lifestyles, and goals than philosophy. She illustrated this opinion zestfully and left me convinced of the subjective nature of the choice we make in finding that one philosophy, rather than another, offers a better description of the world and of the values we hold. The following chapters of this book reveal the basic validity of Goldstein's description. As an experimental biophysicist evaluating noninvasive brain studies, my scientific values had been created by the traditional empirical-inductive scientific methods of hypothesis and observation. It is my philosophical choice to stand by this method and to avoid other philosophical frames for conducting my work. I find certain schools of philosophy and psychology sympathetic to my views of how to think about the brain and its relation to behavior.

The following chapters are written for scientists who are seeking to reflect upon how they compose and interpret neuroimaging experiments studying aspects of behavior. They might appeal to neuroscientists, cognitive scientists, psychologists, philosophers of mind, philosophers of science, and general readers interested in contemporary brain research. Furthermore, since this book touches upon the reliability and limitations of functional imaging methods that are being claimed to offer scientifically objective answers to issues in psychology, economics, linguistics, political sciences, and bioethics, and in the law courts, the book's questioning of what are sometimes considered to be "obvious" truths about the brain should have general implications for a readership beyond these directly interested groups.

CHAPTERS TO COME

Chapter 1 follows up on the questions posed in this introduction about whether mental processes can be explained by neural activities. My concerns about some approaches to localize everyday activities within regions of the brain are examined in terms of the underlying epistemology. The limitations of these efforts are discussed from the viewpoint of a philosophy of Pragmatism, which proposes that words like "working memory" and "consciousness" are abstract concepts that are used to describe the everyday world, but their values for empirically based scientific investigation are yet to be established. For Pragmatism, the meaning of such concepts is determined by the actions they lead to and therefore depends upon their context where their contributions can be assessed.

Regarding neuroscience as a biophysical field, in which physical understanding is sought of biological phenomena, Chapter 2 shows that generalizations in neuroscience are but one example of how untested assumptions proposed to explain human functions are moving physical science away from its empirical-inductive method.

Chapter 3 has selected features from the history of philosophy relevant to neuroimaging, intending to make them accessible to a non-philosopher. Some histories of the qualities of mental processes, assumed and interpreted since Descartes and Galileo, continue to influence contemporary neuroscience. The chapter reviews epistemological assertions about the nature of living processes that were recognized by the great nineteenth-century physiologists who first systematically applied physical science to bodily functions. It is intended to contextualize the assumptions that undergird a scientist's approach to research by reflections on issues that affect scientific choices. This chapter emphasizes the value for neuroscience of philosophical Pragmatism, which, because it denies the value of many traditional philosophical conceptualizations, has been called "less a philosophy than a method of doing without philosophy."[9]

Chapter 4 describes the degree of subjectivity and objectivity in scientific examples and begins to address the general interdisciplinary question of relating subjective phenomena, like human awareness, to objective understanding obtained by physics or chemistry. Niels Bohr faced questions raised about the meaning of the term "electron" by the uncertainty principle. In his *Theory of Complementarity* the description of an electron is complete when we specify how it was measured both as a wave and as a particle, which are subjectively chosen experiments, without integrating these measurements into an "electron" with simultaneous values of velocity and position that can be "objectively" communicated.[10] I propose a neuroscientific analogue in which the fullest available understanding of mental processes is found by simultaneously accepting and correlating experimental observations of human behavior and neurophysiological measurements without trying to unify them into a brain performance of a mental process. Just as the phenomena of an "electron" has lost its usefulness at the quantum level, so too (I propose) have descriptions of mental processes, like "mind," "memory," and "attention," lost their usefulness as explanations at the neuronal level. Long-established concepts like "electron" or "mind," which have been so useful in their respective domains that they have seemed to be innately understood, can no longer be meaningfully discussed in quantum physics or neuroscience, respectively. As Bohr observed, "It is wrong to think that the task of physics is to find out how nature is. Physics concerns what we can say about nature."[11] This scientific approach has been systematized by the philosophy of Mechanisms, recently formalized by Carl Craver,[12] which proposes that an understanding can be created by the many mechanisms found at the different levels that participate in the phenomenon without trying to integrate them.

Chapter 5 reviews neurophysiological measurements and shows how modern neuroimaging methods have become the working tools of brain science by their ability to localize the metabolism of brain energetics and neural firing. This chapter traces the development of these neurophysiological methods for measuring blood flow and the energetics of metabolism, culminating in reproducible, localized, energetic responses to sensory stimulations of animals and humans. The proposals by Cognitive Neuroscience to extend these findings of brain localization to complex mental processes involving subjective, personal responses are analyzed in two typical experimental programs—*willed action* and *working memory*—showing how interpretations continue to be based on hopes of defining these terms in face of experimental disappointments.

Chapter 6 describes our present understanding as to how brain energy consumption is almost completely dedicated to the work of neural firing, as revealed by noninvasive fMRI, MRS, and PET experiments. This leads to an explanation of the metabolic processes responsible for producing the imaging signals. The incremental energies measured during fMRI differencing experiments and the high baseline energy consumption from PET and MRS experiments provide a unified bottom-up understanding of brain activities that allows us to move upward to the higher level of observable behaviors, as discussed in the following chapters.

Earlier chapters have been anticipating the detailed results discussed in Chapter 7 that relate the state of consciousness to physical measurements of brain activity. The approach in this chapter follows the distinction between the *state of* consciousness, which enables the person to respond, and the *acts of* consciousness, discussed in the next chapter, which are the person's specific response to stimuli. Instead of defining consciousness as a mental process, a person is defined to be in the state of consciousness by his ability to respond to simple stimuli. A high level of brain energy production and consumption, evenly distributed throughout the cortex, is shown to be necessary for a person to be in the state of consciousness. A severe reduction of the total energy consumption causes the loss of consciousness during deep anesthesia, slow-wave sleep, or coma.

The acts of consciousness are defined in Chapter 8 as a person knowing that something is of a certain nature and not otherwise. An fMRI BOLD comparison is an example of the acts of consciousness. In a task where the subject is aware of the difference between upside-down and right-side-up faces, or is conscious of either the horizontal or vertical lines in a test of binocular awareness, an fMRI difference signal is clearly observed. These acts of consciousness, together with the total brain energy support of the state of consciousness, create a model of brain function in which individually measured brain activities support identifiable aspects of the person's behavior. These results support a model of brain function in which the person's interests determine brain activity rather than the model of Cognitive Neuroscience in which intrinsic brain properties create human behavior. They show connections between reliable bottom-up brain studies and observable behavior without making psychological assumptions about mental activities.

The epilogue, Chapter 9, reviews autobiographical events that illustrate my intermingled activities in science and the humanities. Acknowledging the powers of science, this story emphasizes the similarities of the two fields rather than focusing on their palpable differences of subject matter and the differing degrees of reliability. Both disciplines are considered to have been built by humans in their effort to understand the world and have relied on the creation and testing of hypotheses as viewed from the perspective of Pragmatism.

NOTES

1. Lauterbur, P. C. (1973). Image formation by induced interactions: Examples employing nuclear magnetic resonance. *Nature, 242*, 190–191.
2. Ogawa, S., Tank, D. W., Menon, R., Ellerman, J. M., Kim, S. G., Merkle, H., & Ugurbil, K. (1992). Intrinsic signal changes accompanying sensory stimulation: functional brain mapping with magnetic resonance imaging. *Proceedings of the National Academy of Sciences USA, 89*, 5951–5955.
3. Kwong, K. K., Belliveau, J. W., Chesler, D. A., Goldberg, I. E., Weiskoff, R. M., Poncelet, B. P., Kennedy, D. N., Hoppel, B. E., Cohen, M. S., Turner, R., Cheng, H. M., Brady, T. J., & Rosen, B. R. (1992). Dynamic magnetic resonance imaging of human brain activity during primary sensory stimulation. *Proceedings of the National Academy of Sciences USA, 89*, 5675–5679.
4. Ogawa, S., Lee, T. M., Kay, A. R., & Tank, D. W. (1990). Brain magnetic resonance imaging with contrast dependent on blood oxygenation. *Proceedings of the National Academy of Sciences USA, 24*, 9868–9872.
5. Phelps, M. E., Huang, S. C., Hoffman, E. J., Selin, C., Sokoloff, L., & Kuhl, D. E. (1979). Tomographic measurement of local cerebral glucose metabolic rate in humans with (F-18)2-fluoro-2-deoxy-D-glucose: validation of method. *Annal of Neurology, 6*(5), 371–388.
6. For a comprehensive account of the application of MRS to the determination of brain energetics and their relation to brain function, see R. G. Shulman & D. L. Rothman

(2004). *Brain energetics & neuronal activity: Applications to fMRI and medicine.* Chichester: John Wiley & Sons.

7. Shulman, R. G., Hyder, F., & Rothman, D. L. (2002). Biophysical basis of brain activity: Implications for neuroimaging. *Q. Rev. Biophys, 35*(3), 287–325.

8. Watson, J. B. (1932). *Behaviorism* (3, 327). New York: Encyclopedia Britannica.

9. Papini, G. (1907). What pragmatism is like (trans. Katherine Royce). *Popular Science Monthly, 71*(4), 351–358, on pages 353–354.

10. Bohr, N. (1987). *The philosophical writings of Niels Bohr, Vol. III, Essays 1958–1962 on atomic physics and human knowledge* (p. 10). Woodbridge, CT: Oxbow Press.

11. Petersen, A. (1963). Philosophy of Niels Bohr. *Bulletin of Atomic Scientists, 19*(7), 8–14.

12. Craver, C. F. (2007). *Explaining the brain: Mechanisms and the mosaic unity of neuroscience.* New York: Oxford University Press.

1

Mind and Matter

Recent advances in imaging have encouraged neuroscientists to investigate a wide range of previously unanswerable questions about brain function. Scientists from the many disciplines of neuroscience—psychology, computer science, linguistics, neurochemistry, and cognition—are designing imaging experiments intended to explore their views of brain activities. Because the images measure glucose and oxygen consumption and the rate of blood flow that supplies these nutrients, the experiments track the traditional physiological parameters of brain energy consumption and metabolism. However, the experimental possibility of measuring changes in brain properties during behavior such as the response to cognitive tasks, sensory stimulation, and the remembrance of events and instructions has encouraged studies of mental processes via these techniques. Views of mental processes are diverse, and I will propose that introducing them as goals of physiological study raises questions about reliability that generally are considered settled matters in physical chemistry. For example, if I want to talk about my forgetfulness with my wife, as in, "My memory is failing! I forgot that I was supposed to play poker last night," our shared sense of the concept of "memory" is very useful for our communication. However, modern imaging experiments raise the question as to whether experiments designed to measure rates of glucose consumption that occur during what the investigator defines as a "memory" task are going to produce results that are as reliable as biochemical experiments that measure glucose incorporation into glycogen. Questions about the meaningfulness of the different kinds of experiments allowed by imaging chemical reactions in the body can be illustrated by comparing two recent applications of these methods.

Note: Chapter 1 was previously published (in essentially the same form) in *Frontiers in Neuroenergetics.*

PHYSICAL STUDIES OF DIABETES

Studies of type 2 diabetes and the brain responses during a memory task both measure chemical reactions of glucose (a common source of human energy), but these different explorations interpret this information very differently. Type 2 diabetes has been around and its properties have been observed for thousands of years. The great Indian physician Sushruta (fl. sixth century BCE) identified the disease[1] and characterized it by ants being attracted to the urine of patients. Now, after 2,000 years of study, we identify the disease by the patient's high blood glucose and by his slow return to normal blood sugar levels after a glucose infusion. We know of the damages wrought by the high glucose, and recent studies using MRS have shown how its immediate cause is downregulation of the insulin control of glucose flow into muscle glycogen.[2] These metabolic results are one step in the growing understanding of this disease. Our scientific understanding uncovers layers of observables—from the sweet smell that once identified the disease to the present biochemical mechanisms contributing to the high blood glucose level. There is in this typical research history not a single step but an unveiling of mechanisms that with time have moved the field of enquiry to the molecular level. Because of these new methods employed in the chemical research—better lenses, really—we now understand the biochemical conditions that cause the disease, and this understanding allows us to control its symptoms. It is now becoming possible to explain this disease at a molecular or cellular level because its defining properties were, from the very beginning of its history, observable and measurable. The story of our unfolding analysis, understanding, and control of type 2 diabetes based on study of its observable properties is one of the triumphs of the scientific method.

METHODS FOR BRAIN STUDIES

The road to understanding brain anatomy and activity has, like our path to understanding diabetes, been much traveled, with advances made possible by methodological and technological advances. Long before the nineteenth-century insights by physiologists, and the subsequent elaboration of neurons, axons, and synapses, we have records from the beginning of the sixteenth century, when, for a brief period, autopsies were allowed in Florence. Leonardo, whose continuing interests in brain anatomy had been interrupted by a temporary ban on the study of cadavers, returned to study the brain's ventricles. Studies of peripheral nerve connections to the ventricles since Galen's time had been inconclusive because the ventricles collapsed when the brain drained upon being excised. Leonardo's beautiful drawings of the preserved ventricles were made possible by casting techniques he brought with him from his ambitious plans for a horse statue.[3] He filled the ventricles with a soft wax that flowed at a warm temperature and solidified when the temperature was lowered. The cast of the brain provided by this innovative method disproved the existence of neuronal connections to the ventricles that had been believed for more than 1,000 years.

Today, in conjunction with other approaches in neuroscience, progress in brain studies is being fueled by the chemical and metabolic information provided by noninvasive imaging methods. Noninvasive methods of fMRI, MRS, and PET are responsible for our growing ability to look into the complexities of brain chemistry and physics.

Measurements of the cerebral flow of blood and metabolism showed that the brain obtained energy and synthesized metabolic products by oxidizing glucose. These noninvasive methods, in conjunction with other approaches, have made it possible to measure and localize cerebral metabolites, thereby allowing us to directly follow metabolism in humans. These developments have created a wide range of possible directions for neuroscience. With regard to biochemical understanding, the metabolic studies of the brain provide data at the molecular level from similar experiments as those that are responsible for our present understanding of type 2 diabetes. But armed with these new tools, neuroimaging research has also turned to studying mental processes like "memory" or "consciousness." There are thousands of reports on efforts to localize the brain regions responsible for mental processes whose origins are to be found in many disciplines, particularly psychology, although rapidly being extended to the social sciences like economics, law, and political science.

This book will focus on the similarities and differences of scientific method between these two kinds of studies—of the metabolism responsible for diabetes and of the brain participation in mental processes. While it will focus on noninvasive investigations of brain function and metabolism, it is also a more basic story of how we posit and pursue questions in scientific research. It is about observation and our ability to make limited assertions—meaning that it is meant to be a celebration of what we can accomplish in the conduct of observation, experimentation, and analysis, and the risks of an alternate method: of allowing *a priori* assumptions to have undue influence on the conduct of our science. I will ask how we have gone from measurements of brain chemistry to assertions about the mind, and whether chemistry should seek to explain such concepts.

MY PATH INTO NEUROSCIENCE

As a biophysicist I have been enthusiastic about physical studies that can reveal the molecular or cellular mechanism of biological processes—that is what biophysicists and physiologists do. The achievements of physiology testify to the successes of this method: the energy consumption of muscle work, the circulation of blood, and the understanding of diseases provide explanations and opportunities for control at the molecular level. The surging discoveries in molecular biology supported by novel noninvasive techniques for studying brain activities have encouraged neuroscientists to add brain function and psychological processes to the topics that can be studied at the molecular level. The question for the practicing scientist becomes, "What are the criteria for selecting biological phenomena that can be studied with the expectation of finding explanations at the physical-chemical level?" I have come to my own answers about these questions only after decades of research, and some notable wrong turns.

I had been doing magnetic research since the 1950s and in the early 1990s, when, using MRS to study neurophysiology, I took an excursion offered by the discovery of fMRI,[4,5] which showed that localized changes in brain activity in response to sensory stimulation, such as shining light in the eyes, could be detected. Soon after Seiji Ogawa's demonstration of fMRI with Kamil Ugurbil, both he and Kamil, former colleagues at Bell Labs, came to our Yale laboratory to extend their original measurements on our NMR equipment, which Andrew Blamire and Douglas Rothman had modified so as to do fMRI experiments.[6]

At this time the field was ablaze as reports accumulated of fMRI responses to various stimuli in numerous laboratories, including reports of brain activities during cognitive tasks like remembering a room or executing a numerical task. In that heady atmosphere, where it seemed that mysteries of the mind, activities such as memory and consciousness, were being revealed as regional brain activations, I asked a knowledgeable colleague what well-established mental activity we could study on our equipment where we had already measured brain responses to light. My colleague, Patricia Goldman-Rakic, suggested that since short-term memory (sometimes called "working memory") had been identified by invasive electrodes in a specific brain region in nonhuman primates, we might look for an analogous response in the human brain. The reigning psychological paradigm of Cognitive Neuroscience assumed that a particular region would be specifically and exclusively motivated by a single activity—in the case at hand, working memory. We did the experiment and found that a particular frontal region indeed was active when the person was doing a task that required short-term remembering, and we published the results.[7]

However, in the excitement of finding a localized brain response to a psychological concept, we had been too excited to subject the important claims of Cognitive Neuroscience to the crucial test of whether the localized response was unique. Our subsequent, more careful, controlled experiments showed that the same region was activated when the subject merely paid attention to a stimulus that did not require remembering.[8] These results, which tested the assumption that there was a unique region responding to what was called "working memory," contradicted that psychological model. The upshot of these experiments was that the same region was activated during a task requiring attention (and many other activities) without the person being required to remember an earlier event.[9] Since the regional activation was not a sufficient response to remembering as postulated by Cognitive Neuroscience, it seemed necessary to unpack the assumptions and findings of Cognitive Neuroscience in order to understand what brain activity could tell us about psychological activities. The results of this endeavor, proposed in 1996,[8] are summarized in this book.

These experiments and subsequent studies helped me to realize that we had inadvertently launched experiments without reflecting upon the way in which we were working within our normal life—the "I didn't remember that I had a poker game last night" sort of assumptions. Because we were keen to use physical measurements to identify psychological processes in the brain, we assumed that we knew what those processes were. When studying metabolism and energetics, as in the synthesis of glycogen in diabetes, it had not been necessary to reexamine epistemological assumptions about the scientific method. However, in studying topics like working memory, we were not just seeking to measure metabolic responses to clearly defined sensory stimulations by light, sound, or odors; we sought to look at activities of the mind. Like many others, I was eager to locate brain activities that supported our mental life. But as our experiments showed, "working memory" was not being located in the physiological world that we could measure empirically. Instead it was driven by an assumption, a hypothesis about brain activity—a hypothesis that was not supported by the experiments. Our enthusiasm was widely shared; our results were typical of experimental reports in this active field, in that neuroimaging experiments had been failing to identify unique brain locations supporting mental concepts.[9-11] Most directly these results raised the question as to how studies of mental processes differ from scientific investigations capable of explaining more material processes such as type 2 diabetes.

POWERS AND LIMITS OF PHYSICAL EXPLANATIONS

From the early empirical refining of metals to today's understanding and control of manmade materials, we can trace the advances in the physical and chemical understanding of nonliving phenomenon. The highly developed understanding of the inorganic world has continuously been extended to the living world of plants and animals, including humans. Our subject is part of this great historical movement in which studies are broadening to explain the physics and chemistry involved in human phenomenon such as health and behavior. Given the rapid progress in modern biological research directions such as generated by genetics, computer data handling, and brain imaging, it is difficult to imagine what limits exist on the understanding that can rightfully be expected from biophysical research.

When we come to the issue at hand, as to how far physics and chemistry can explain the workings of the human brain, we can profit from the analyses offered by history. The excitement felt today is a continuation of the innovative experiments in the nineteenth century by Claude Bernard and Hermann von Helmholtz, who laid the foundations of today's physiology. Bernard proposed methods for physical and chemical explanations of bodily processes by insisting that the object of scientific research "is the same for living bodies as for inorganic bodies; it consists in finding the relations that connect any phenomenon with its immediate cause, or putting it differently, it consists in finding the conditions necessary for the appearance of the phenomenon."[12] To identify these connections Bernard proposed that phenomena be disassociated into simpler phenomena until finding conditions that cannot be analyzed further in the present state of science: in other words, into chemical or physical processes or mechanisms. The goal was to discover the necessary chemical or physical mechanism that caused a phenomenon, and in this way we would understand as well as possible how processes occurred. However, he continued, "The nature of our minds leads us to seek the essence or the *why* of things. Thus we aim beyond the goal that it is given us to reach; for experience soon teaches us that we cannot get beyond the *how*,i.e.,beyond the immediate cause or the necessary conditions of phenomena. In this respect the limits of our knowledge are the same in biological as in physical-chemical sciences."[13]

In neuroscience, brain activities are traditionally disassociated into elementary electrical, chemical, and structural processes. When brain activity is described at the electrochemical level of ion movements across membranes or at the physical level of energy consumption, it is, for the present purposes, not reducible further, because the chemical fluxes of ions and brain energy are (in today's science) the ultimate explanations in chemical-physical terms—the hope of biological explanations. To reach this resting point where no further breakdown is needed, we have to decompose the general description of activities attributed to the brain into these components. Thus we can find the conditions necessary for the phenomenon of brain activity to take place. We have reached the ultimate in understanding brain activity when it is expressed in its different components of action potentials and energy consumption that can be described in measurable chemical terms. That understanding is not of the original descriptions of the phenomenon, which was the kind of brain activity that could be identified by lesions or neuroimages, but it was that activity reduced to more physically explainable mechanisms. To describe how a phenomenon happens at the physical-chemical level is the goal of the starting observations. The conditions that are necessary for the phenomenon to occur explain *how* it happens, and additional studies at the electrochemical level can amplify our understanding by connecting it with other physical processes, but they do not describe why it happens. When we try to describe *why* something happens, we are hoping to have understood it at a deeper level, where the explanation is complete and is uniquely responsible for the event. In arguing that we cannot go beyond physicochemical explanations, Bernard was addressing the vitalist's views that there were fundamental forces such as the *élan vital* whose explanatory powers provided a more fundamental explanation of why bodily processes occurred. In denying the possibility of explaining why something happens, Bernard was fighting a recurrent position in history. Newton's laws of gravity were dismissed by some philosophers in his day as having merely written Kepler's laws in terms of mathematical equations, and were criticized for not having provided an explanation of *why* two bodies attracted each other with a force of gravity.

In looking for an explanation of human behavior by brain processes, I will argue that we should remember that we too are limited to the physical. Physical experiments can find necessary explanations of how things happen at the chemical or physical level, but they cannot justify these explanations by appealing to a higher authority because there is no empirically sound basis for concepts that proffer higher authority than physical and chemical explanations. When brain activations are attributed to psychologically postulated mental processes such as consciousness, memory, or intention instead of describing physical-chemical brain activities that occur when the person is performing the observed behavior, these experimental results are presumed to tell us *why* the individual responds to stimuli, or remembers or intends to perform an act. It is possible to find brain activities necessary for an observable human performance: a functioning medial temporal lobe is necessary for a person to remember events and, as we shall see, a high level of brain energy consumption is needed for a person to be in a state of consciousness. On the other hand, by postulating that a mental activity called "working memory" is the cause of a person remembering something, we are setting aside the need for a connection between observables (a particular prefrontal brain region becomes more active when the person is performing a particular act) for a theory of mental activities that cause the chemical actions. Abstract concepts do not carry discrete causal powers.

PRAGMATISM AND THE MEANING OF WORDS

As any scientist takes on a research question, he or she functions (consciously or not) within a set of methodological assumptions. My point in the preceding section was that I, along with many other brain scientists, unconsciously drifted from the traditional views of an epistemology that was limited to empirical observable experiments into a realm that transferred "everyday" assumptions about mental acts into research. Some scientists may well feel that such concepts **are** clear and distinct enough to shape an experiment, and certainly many non-scientists who are hoping that neuroscience can throw light on crime, economic behavior, or reactions to art are likely to unconsciously subscribe to an epistemology that grants significance to such abstract concepts. But in justifying constraining our ambitions when reflecting upon our epistemology, there are other philosophers who caution us about the use of abstract words— proposing that words have meaning only to the extent they influence action. These Pragmatists advise us not to assume we actually understand something simply because we have a word for it.

The Pragmatist philosopher Williams James wrote how it is a mistake to look to words to help understand mysteries:[14]

> You know how men have always hankered after unlawful magic, and you know what a great art, in magic, WORDS have always played, If you have his name or the formula of incantation that binds him you can control the spirit, genie, a friete, or whatever the power may be.
>
> ...So the universe has always appeared to the natural mind as a kind of enigma. Of which the key must be sought in the shape of (an) illuminating or power-bringing word or name. That word names the universe's PRINCIPLE and to possess it is, after a fashion, to possess, the universe itself. "God," "Matter," "Reason," "The Absolute," "Energy," are so many solving names. You can rest when you have them. You are [at] the end of your metaphysical quest. But if you follow the pragmatic method, you cannot look on any such word as closing your quest. You must bring out of each word its practical cash-value, see it at work within the stream of your experience. It appears less as a solution, than as a program for more work,

and more particularly as an indication of the ways in which existing realities may be CHANGED. [Italics and capitalization are James's.]

What I understand James to be saying is that the existence of a word doesn't solidify a concept. He was talking about theology, but in a very similar vein, I would suggest that we have not defined "truth" or "memory" just because we have words for them. A concept like "working memory" is defined by the actions it leads to and therefore is intrinsically dependent upon its specific usage or the context in which it is identified. When we claim working memory is found in a person who is remembering recently observed numbers or faces or the third-to-last word he saw, we are not starting with the observation of a general property found in all cases, like the sweet smell of urine identifying diabetes, but are proposing there is a general concept that underlies all these observations. We can profitably use a word like "memory" to describe how well something is remembered by a person or group (or whether I am habitually forgetting my poker dates), but it is a long stretch to assume that the word "memory" used to describe a student reciting the multiplication table is the same thing as the word Marcel Proust used to describe what was evoked by the smell of madeleines. It is difficult to see how reliably identical brain activities might be found for such a word. And, in fact, experimental fMRI results do not find a single reproducible response for a term such as "working memory" but rather find different brain responses that depend upon the context in which the term is used.[9-11] These results are in agreement with the Pragmatist's view that there is no substance to the word other than in the actions it generates.

Why do I claim that biological processes like the immune response, genetics, and metabolism can be explained in physical-chemical terms while mental processes like memory and consciousness cannot be? The simple answer is that inheritance of traits, the immune response, and metabolism are activities that can be observed and measured while the psychological processes described as memory or intentions are not observables but are hypotheses created by theories that help us describe the world.

FRANCIS CRICK'S STUDY OF CONSCIOUSNESS

The distinction in neuroscience between experiments designed to reduce conceptualizations of biological phenomena to molecules and cells and experiments designed to find molecular and cellular mechanisms of observables can be seen clearly in the studies of the abstraction called consciousness. Consciousness is a central interest today of neuroscientists, attracting discussions from its many subdisciplines. Journals, books, associations, and an annual meeting all specifically address the study of consciousness.

It may come as no surprise that the search for a molecular basis of consciousness has been led by Francis Crick, whose great elucidation of the DNA structure led to the field of molecular biology, the twentieth-century revolution in biology. In 1994 Crick focused the study of consciousness when in his book *The Astonishing Hypothesis: The Scientific Search for the Soul*,[15] he stated: "our minds—the behavior of our brains—can be explained by the interactions of nerve cells (and other cells) and the molecules associated with them" (p. 7). Crick defines the terms of his reductionist approach in this way: "a complex system can be explained by the behavior of its parts," and he proposes that the reduction needs to go no further than finding explanations at the neural or chemical level using the laws of classical physics.

In advocating the explanation of consciousness at the neural level, he writes that such reductionism is "not the rigid processes of explaining one set of ideas in terms of another fixed set of ideas at a lower level, but a dynamic interactive process that modifies the concepts at both levels as the knowledge develops."[16] He recognizes that since Descartes the mental and the material have been considered to be separate, incommensurate domains, but claims that this method of explaining a system property at the chemical level does not involve a "category mistake." He acknowledges that the mental and material have been considered to be of different categories and that proposing to explain one in terms of the other has been considered to be a mistake (the familiar body–mind problem), but he claims that recent advances in reductionist studies have enabled science to overcome these categorical differences. In support of this hypothesis, he notes that in earlier days the problem of a reductionist approach "could have taken the form that to consider a gene to be a molecule (or as we should say now, a part of a matched pair of molecules) would be a category mistake. A gene is one category and a molecule is a quite different category. One can see now how hollow such objections have turned out to be."[17] In my opinion, this statement, made in the optimistic early days of the Human Genome Project asserting that the DNA molecule explained the gene, is misleading in two important ways.

First, Crick proposes that the gene that has been explained by DNA is of the same category as consciousness and thereby sets an example for his goal to reduce consciousness to molecules. However, the gene, at the beginning of Crick and Watson's studies, had been defined by observations as the fundamental unit of inheritance.[18] The properties of genes were observables: Mendel's pea shoots reflected genes for yellow or green peas, while the genes identified in Morgan's fruit flies controlled the inheritance of red eyes and other observable traits. In this important respect the gene differed from consciousness, which Crick acknowledged could not be defined by observation. The explication of the DNA structure provides a way to study the processes of inheritance attributed to the gene in molecular terms. The DNA structure became the basis of a new field of study, molecular genetics, which will continue the study of the many steps of inheritance (e.g., meiosis, development, and phenotype expression) in molecular terms.[19] In this role DNA actually serves as the beginning of biochemical research into the processes of heredity. The observable inheritance of many physical properties, like the red eye in Drosophila, now can be explained at the molecular level starting with the DNA sequence just as the observable sweet smell identifying diabetes now can be explained by the metabolism of glucose. But consciousness is not an observable: it was a concept presumed to underlie a person's behavior. It was of a different category than the gene, and there is no reason to believe that advances in biology have suddenly made it understandable in molecule terms. Hence, the role of DNA in providing mechanisms for actions attributed to the gene is very different from how Crick proposes to explain that "You, your joys and your sorrows and your ambitions, your sense of personal identity and free will are in fact no more than the behavior of a vast assembly of nerve cells and their associated molecules."[20]

My second criticism is that Francis Crick and Jim Watson never studied the gene, although their results have important consequences for understanding the process of heritability. They studied base pairing, hydrogen bonds, x-ray diffraction patterns, and possible structural models of the DNA molecule. Their structural studies of a chemical molecule that had been known to be involved in genetic processes changed our understanding of genetics and biology for all time—but they didn't study the gene. Although the gene was a description of the observable processes of inheritance, those processes had not been described in molecular terms and could not be studied directly. When Crick suggests that molecular studies are a useful method for explaining consciousness, he is asking us to do something quite different from what he and Watson did.

In brain studies I suggest we should do what Crick and Watson actually did, not what Crick subsequently proposed. They studied the properties of a molecule that previously had been shown to play a necessary role in the observable transmission of genetic information and thereby opened observable, inheritable traits, like the red eyes of Drosophila, to molecular studies.

A DIFFERENT APPROACH TO THE STUDY OF CONSCIOUSNESS

A philosophical position that I have found helpful in starting to relate brain function to physical brain studies has been proposed by Maxwell Bennett and

Peter Hacker.[9] Bennett and Hacker criticized a fundamental assumption of Cognitive Neuroscience that localizes mental processes like memory or attention in the brain. They claim that this assertion is conceptually wrong in that "it ascribes to the brain attributes that it makes sense only to ascribe to the animal as a whole." Bennett and Hacker claim this is nonsensical because "the brain cannot be conscious—only the living creature whose brain it is can be conscious—or unconscious."

Bennett and Hacker conclude that the brain does not perform any of the mental functions postulated for it—it does not do memory or make decisions. Their position that brain activity supports the person's behavior is quite the opposite of the view in Cognitive Neuroscience that brain activity causes behavior. Bennett and Hacker note that an active, healthy brain is necessary for a person's behavior such as remembering or deciding. A normal medial temporal lobe is necessary for the person to remember something from long ago just as a healthy motor cortex is needed for the person to perform acts of physical dexterity. Brain activity, in this view, supports the person who has the thoughts and performs the actions. In accepting this view I propose to show how experimental measurements of brain energy are explicitly dedicated to supporting definable features of human behavior.

Because of the differing capabilities of neuroimaging methods, the parameters of total and incremental brain energy consumption are measured and reported separately. The following pages show, by combining MRS and PET measurements of total brain energy consumption, that a very large fraction (~80%) of brain energy supports neural firing in the absence of intentional stimuli, or, as it called, in the resting state.[11] In contrast to this dominant use of energy, fMRI measurements show small energy changes induced by stimuli. These incremental energies ranged from a maximum of ~15% during intense sensory stimulation to less than 1% during cognitive tasks.

In following the successes carved out by Crick and Watson, I propose that to explore consciousness we should first define consciousness by observable behavior and then find physical brain activities that are properties of the person showing that behavior. This approach should increasingly reveal the nature of brain mechanisms supporting a person in the observable state of consciousness—just as the studies of the DNA structure revealed mechanisms that described inheritance. We have proposed how this can be done in a preliminary report[21] sketching a study that related high brain energy to the person's state of consciousness that was defined by behavior—by the person's responses to simple stimuli. The state of consciousness defines a condition where the person is conscious or awake as opposed to being unconscious or asleep. There is no mystery or contingency in saying that a person is in a state of consciousness when we see him responding to simple questions or touches—anesthesiologists do it all the time, and their conclusion is the basis of important clinical decisions. Once a person can be defined as being in the state of consciousness by observing his response to stimuli, we can measure properties of that state, including brain activities. We have identified brain properties characteristic of that state that decrease substantially when the person loses consciousness—as a result of anesthesia or falling asleep or suffering a coma. Experiments from MRS and PET, reviewed in the following pages, show that the high global level of neural energy plays a necessary role in maintaining humans in the observable, behavioral state of consciousness. Hence, these results establish a connection between total, global neural activity and the observable state of consciousness and open the neural properties of that state to further molecular study.

The second aspect of consciousness, called the acts of consciousness, consists of the person's ability to recognize and decide upon things—to know that they are of a particular meaning rather than of an alternative. The acts of consciousness are commonly observed during fMRI experiments where the incremental brain activities are measured as the subject responds to the difference between two conditions. When the person is knowledgeable about the difference in the two conditions, such as during sensory stimulation, brain responses are discrete localized, and reproducible, whereas when the differences are less well defined, such as during "working memory" comparisons, the brain responses are less well localized and depend on the context. The reason for the differences in brain responses to these two kinds of stimuli has been a recurring question in neuroimaging studies. I propose that the first condition needed to explain why some brain responses are very well localized and others not is that the brain is active in support of the person's interests rather than having intrinsic, built-in activities. The second requirement for a discrete reproducible brain response to the person's activities is that such activities must be clearly defined. For a Pragmatist, sensory stimuli give reproducible brain responses because the stimuli themselves are well defined, whereas the brain response to abstract concepts is not reproducible because such concepts are not clearly defined. As a result of following these philosophical approaches, reliable physical studies of cerebral energetics and work can be extended to establish correlations with human behavior. Evidence for these views is presented in the later chapters. To appreciate these findings, we first review the understanding of neuronal energy consumption and work that has been created by neuroimaging experiments and evaluate competing models of brain function that propose to relate these physical measurements to behavior.

NOTES

1. Lock, S., et al. (2001). *The Oxford illustrated companion to medicine* (p. 420). New York: Oxford University Press.
2. Shulman, R. G., & Rothman, D. L. (2001). ^{13}C NMR of intermediary metabolism: Implications for systemic physiology. *Ann Rev Physiol, 63,* 15–48.
3. da Vinci, L. (1992). *The anatomy of man: Drawings from the collection of Her Majesty Queen Elizabeth II.* Boston, Toronto, London: Museum of Fine Arts Houston and Bullfinch Press, Little Brown & Co.
4. Ogawa, S., Tank, D. W., Menon, R., Ellerman, J. M., Kim, S. G., Merkle, H., & Ugurbil, K. (1992). Intrinsic signal changes accompanying sensory stimulation: functional brain mapping with magnetic resonance imaging. *Proceedings of the National Academy of Sciences USA, 89,* 5951–5955.
5. Kwong, K. K., Belliveau, J. W., Chesler, D. A., Goldberg, I. E., Weiskoff, R. M., Poncelet, B. P., Kennedy, D. N., Hoppel, B. E., Cohen, M. S., Turner, R., Cheng, H. M., Brady, T. J., & Rosen, B. R. (1992). Dynamic magnetic resonance imaging of human brain activity during primary sensory stimulation. *Proceedings of the National Academy of Sciences USA, 89,* 5675–5679.
6. Blamire, A. M., Ogawa, S., Ugurbil, K., Rothman, D. L., McCarthy, G., Ellerman, J. M., Hyder, F., Rattner, Z., & Shulman, R. G. (1992). Dynamic mapping of the human visual cortex by high-speed magnetic resonance imaging. *Proceedings of the National Academy of Sciences USA, 89*(22), 11069–11073.
7. McCarthy, G., Blamire, A. M., Puce, A., Nobre, A. C., Bloch, G., Hyder, F., Goldman-Rakic, P., & Shulman, R. G. (1994). Functional magnetic resonance imaging of human prefrontal cortex activation during a spatial working memory task. *Proceedings of the National Academy of Sciences USA, 91*(18), 8690–8694.
8. Shulman, R. G. (1996). An interview with Robert G. Shulman. *J Cogn Neurosci, 8*(5), 474–480.
9. Shulman, R. G., Hyder, F., & Rothman, D. L. (2002). Biophysical basis of brain activity: Implications for neuroimaging. *Q Rev Biophys, 35*(3), 287–325.
10. Fodor, J. (2000). *The mind doesn't work that way: The scope and limits of computational psychology.* Cambridge, MA: MIT Press. Fodor, an early contributor to cognitive psychology, abandoned the theory because neuroimaging results had shown that brain responses were not modular and depended upon context. Therefore, he concluded the brain did not act in a logical manner as a Turing computer and neuroimaging was an empirical subject. In discussing how and why the model of a computer-like brain is not working, I echo Fodor's argument. This book emphasizes that neuroimaging results are not modular in order to take advantage of the great promise they have for creating an empirical brain science.
11. Friston, K. (2009). Modalities, modes and modes in functional neuroimaging. *Science, 326,* 399–403. This summary of Karl Friston's extensive contributions to fMRI allows me to distinguish between my unbounded admiration for fMRI as a method for creating an empirical science and my criticism of claims that fMRI results actually find the modular brain regions proposed by computer theories of brain activity. Friston early on recognized that psychological concepts like working

memory were not being localized to unique brain regions and has conducted an impressive empirical program designed to correct these expectations and to find a use for fMRI in brain function. However, since his SPM computer program is almost universally used in support of modularity, his own work illustrates the ambiguity in the field between disavowing modularity and at the same time hankering after it. I hope that this book illustrates my own admiration for the value of fMRI for empirical studies, which has been carried forward by many wonderful scientific efforts. My appreciation of the empirical work, in addition to the energetics discussed in the text, particularly values the development of techniques and instrumentation for increased sensitivity and the numerous investigations of the fusiform face area, which is an active topic of empirical research.

12. Bernard, C. (1957). *An introduction to the study of experimental medicine* (trans. Henry Copley Greene; p. 66). New York: Dover Publications.
13. Ibid. (p. 80).
14. James, W. (1975). *Pragmatism: A new name for some old ways of thinking* (p.31). Harvard University Press, Cambridge, MA.
15. Crick, F. H. C. (1994). *The astonishing hypothesis.* New York: Charles Scribner's Sons.
16. Ibid. (p. 8).
17. Ibid. (p. 9).
18. Encyclopedia Britannica (1932). Gene. *Encyclopedia Britannica* (14th ed., vol. 10, p. 100). New York.
19. Keller, E. F. (2000). *The century of the gene* (pp. 155–159). Cambridge, MA: Harvard University Press. After showing there is no single definition of the very useful term "gene," the author points out that "One single entity was taken to be the guarantor of intergenerational stability, the factor responsible for individual traits, and, at the same time, the agent directing the organism's development."
20. Crick, op. cit. (p. 3).
21. Shulman, R. G., Hyder, F., & Rothman, D. L. (2009). Baseline brain energy supports the state of consciousness. *Proceedings of the National Academy of Sciences USA, 102*, 11096–11101.

2

Biophysics

An Empirical Science

euroscience is a biophysical field where the explanatory powers of physical science are applied to brain functions. As chemical and biological sciences developed, physical laws were applied to processes of living tissue. Although biology and physics have long been intermingled, the general direction of explanation, of which neuroscience is a contemporary example, has been to extend physical understanding to aspects of biological phenomena. Continuing advances in biophysical understanding, obtained by the empirical, inductive methods developed for physical science, have maintained optimism about the value of these studies.

Physical studies of biomolecules go back at least to Louis Pasteur, who in 1857 used state-of-the-art optical methods to distinguish the two isomers of tartaric acid. He found that although both were formed in chemical reactions, only one was digested by living molds. This discovery led Pasteur to postulate that living organisms selected molecules on the basis of symmetry. Subsequently, when confronted by analogous symmetries that arose during the industrial fermentation of beer by yeast, he concluded that fermentation is a property of living systems. In this early study molecular properties helped answer a major biological question of the day: What chemical reactions distinguish the living from the nonliving? His answer, which provides an early model for our brain studies, is that symmetry was a property of living creatures; it didn't explain life, but it was a reliable characteristic.

At the same time, in Liège, Theodor Schwann was developing the cellular theory of organic life. By showing that the cell was the basic building block of both plant and animal life, he instigated physiological studies of the organism in terms of its cellular components. In the early twentieth century, Santiago Ramón y Cajal identified the cells in the brain that brought that organ into scientific view. Investigation of the structure–function relationships of more and more complex biomolecules culminated in the elucidation of the structure of DNA and hemoglobin in the middle of the last century. These outstanding discoveries, and their subsequent expansions in the past 50 years, underlie our understanding of the molecular bases of fermentation, the integrity of cells, and modern molecular biology. Given the many properties of cells that have now been explained at the molecular level, it is no wonder that the exploration of biological molecules and cells seems to promise ever-expanding understanding of human activities at these higher levels. Yet as we shall see scientific advances are not linear, not progressing smoothly toward better understanding; there are detours, possibly dead ends, created by overenthusiastic claims about the explanatory powers of the physical sciences. The powers of empirical physical approaches to biological phenomena and the risks of moving away from experimental criteria under the influence of biological theories will be described in this chapter. The question addressed herein is not whether physical science can contribute to our understanding of biological processes, but rather how it can best be done.

GOLDEN YEARS

In surveying some of the methods being used in neuroscience, the previous chapter invoked the Pragmatist's warning that the words we use to describe the world were often hypotheses at an early stage of an understanding, not at its conclusion. Hypotheses that rely upon abstract concepts are contingencies whose epistemic value is judged by the actions they lead to. Inferring a hypothesis that is subsequently to be tested is the familiar method of physical science. As experiments continue to prove the usefulness of a hypothesis, it becomes recognized as a law whose applicability can be trusted—for example, when biophysics uses thermodynamics to explain steps of biological processes. I assume that laws from physics and chemistry can be used to reveal and test hypotheses about mechanisms that are necessary for biological phenomena. In this way physical science builds an understanding of the phenomena. However, this is a different goal than assuming that laws can be found that can explain biological phenomena with the same completeness that physics can describe the motions of a billiard ball or of the planets.

The value and nature of physical and chemical explanations of steps contributing to biological phenomena became apparent to me during two decades of research in condensed-matter physics and biophysics at the Bell Telephone Laboratories. Many colleagues were of my age, and the talents and energies of this unruly crowd were guided by a rational scientific management. Administrative decisions were made on the basis of authentic understanding and the resources were distributed to further directions that promised scientific understanding, and only occasionally on the promise of practical applications. Bill Baker, the president of Bell Telephone Laboratories, once said, explaining his support for biophysics research, that while biophysics research is not needed by AT&T, it was needed by Bell Laboratories, and Bell Laboratories, he continued, is undoubtedly needed by AT&T. The need to convert basic research into practical usage was accomplished by the many layers of development, engineering, and production serving the communication goals of the Bell System. In this corporate structure researchers at Bell Laboratories had an unusual degree of freedom to pursue knowledge, and they did so by empirical-inductive methods, the ideal of physical science.

In 1961, while doing research on the physics of semiconductors, superconductors, and magnetic materials, mainly by NMR, I was brought by a series of unplanned events into a study of biological materials. Russian scientists had reported that DNA molecules were magnetic, seemingly embodying a swarm of unpaired electron spins. I obtained some cotton-like threads of DNA and, testing them in an electron spin resonance spectrometer, found that they were indeed magnetic. Our experiments soon showed that the electron spins were ferromagnetic; they were all lined up like the electrons in iron magnets. The hypothesis that DNA electrons were coupled thrilled me with the hope that this unexpected, and unparalleled, physical phenomenon might help explain the mysteries of biology in general and inheritance in particular. I did run around Bell Labs telling all my friends the great news that DNA had unexpected electronic properties, but before publishing the results, it was necessary to make sure that the electrons being measured were really in the DNA molecule, not, for example, in some impurity accompanying the DNA. A few elementary measurements turned up the existence of clumps of ferromagnetic impurities in the samples, little pieces of iron oxides, which further research showed were products of the DNA extraction process. This provided an explanation for the Russian publications, disproving the revolutionary hypothesis indicated by the early data, and allowed our research to proceed in other directions. But it changed my goals; the hook had been set: I had experienced the excitement of biological research. This new direction changed my sabbatical plans at the last moment from condensed-matter physics to molecular biology and biophysics. With the blessings of the Guggenheim Foundation I went to the hut in the courtyard of the Cavendish Laboratory in Cambridge to do research for a year on the reading of the genetic code with Francis Crick and Sidney Brenner. At Cambridge I moved without any biochemical experience into Crick's laboratory to perform bacteriophage experiments, testing his quite abstract theory of how the genetic code was read. In the early 1960s the very existence of a genetic code, let alone its nature, was pure conjecture. Crick's hypothesis was that the sequence of bases in DNA was read as a triplet code where every combination of three nucleotides was the signal for a specific amino acid to be incorporated into a protein. He proposed further that the DNA code was read serially, one triplet at a time, like a magnetic tape. When an acridine molecule, acting as a mutagen, is inserted in the DNA between two adjacent base-paired nucleotides, he proposed it is included by the reading mechanism in a triplet. In the subsequent reading of the DNA each triplet, assumed to code for a specific amino acid, was shifted by one base-pair, resulting in coding for a different amino acid. At a time when the triplet code was only a hypothesis, Crick proposed that a triplet code existed and furthermore he proposed bacteriophage experiments testing the hypothesis about the mechanism by which the code was read. Although the simple experiments I did daily were at the edge of my inexperienced understanding (three drops of this and 1 cc of that into a Petri dish followed by overnight in the oven), the reading model being tested was a grand hypothesis based upon understanding and guesswork. As the results continued to support the hypothesis, Crick, more than once, walked around the lab expressing the fear that the next experiment would disprove the whole structure, so that hypothesis and explanations would be flushed down the drain. But they survived, and the frame-shift reading model remains a foundation of molecular biology.[1]

These examples illustrate the generating powers of a hypothesis, treated deferentially and skeptically in an inductive science based on the fluid interaction of hypothesis and observation. They emphasize the dynamic nature of proposing explanations of a phenomenon that can be abandoned when the hypothesis is disproven or strengthened when it is supported by experiments. Inductive science chooses questions to answer (how is the sequence of amino acids in a protein determined by the DNA sequence?); then proposes a hypothesis for an answer (DNA is read three base-pairs at a time serially, and the introduction of a chemical that looks like a base-pair will cause all downstream triplets to be read incorrectly); then tests this prediction by experiments. After continuing experimental support, the hypothesis determines the next questions to be asked. This procedure is generally recognized as the essence of good science. The process of moving systematically from one issue to the next, while maintaining a creative tension between skepticism and insight, is what makes science so exciting.

Returning to Bell Telephone Labs with an experience of modern biology, my colleagues and I were encouraged by the far-sighted management to continue biophysical research. We studied biological materials (e.g., proteins and nucleic acids) with magnetic resonance methods such as we had previously introduced into physical studies of semiconductors, superconductors, and anti-ferromagnetics. Our approach was similar to that being used by the condensed-matter physicists and chemists who were our colleagues. If you conduct biological research in a laboratory devoted to understanding the physics of molecules and inorganic materials, you must use the methods of physics to study biological materials. Furthermore, it was necessary to use the same criteria to judge the success of that effort. The Bell Labs administration was eager to support research efforts so long as they gave definite results. Our biophysical goals were similar; we accepted that explanations had to be based on established physical principles and that only on that basis could one securely obtain the kind of understanding Bell Labs researchers were seeking. Explanatory mechanisms resulted from the interaction between theory and experiment, between hypothesis and empirical testing and then backward from empiricism to hypothesis. The original quantum mechanical explanations of the simplest materials like the hydrogen atom had been extended to more complex materials like semiconductors of practical interest to the telephone company. The methods were traditionally empirical, but novel questions had to be formulated so as to allow physical solutions.[2]

THOMAS KUHN AND NORMAL SCIENCE

To understand the methods of biophysical research in more general terms, we start with Thomas Kuhn's 1962 essay *The Structure of Scientific Revolutions*,[3] which divided scientific research into periods of normal science and revolutionary science. Kuhn argued that normal science is characterized by generally accepted paradigms that are concepts and methodologies that are useful for answering questions and solving puzzles. Paradigms are hypotheses that are not questioned during this period. Cumulatively, the solutions to these puzzles provide an understanding of nature that, for example, in condensed-matter physics resulted in technological progress. As more and more solutions are found, new questions arise that are unanswerable in the context of the original paradigms. This leads to the need for new concepts with superior explanatory powers that sooner or later generate the new paradigms.

Kuhn originally proposed that changes in the paradigms occurred only during scientific revolutions, when paradigms of normal science are replaced by novel concepts. In this view scientific concepts create revolutions. They are accepted, he proposes, because the older paradigms have run into contradictions, or new data have introduced novel results—or when the new theory offered more satisfactory explanations, such as when atomic physics required explanations that could not be found by classical laws. For Kuhn, whose examples came from the history of physics, the two periods of normal and revolutionary science were rather easily distinguished.

Kuhn's analysis provides a popular starting point for evaluating biophysical research, but because of the differences between biology and physics his distinctions between normal and revolutionary science must be modified, softened to more accurately reflect the biophysical world. For both the normal and revolutionary periods of physics and more urgently for biological research, the structures as originally postulated by Kuhn are too easily distinguished and too static. Recent biophysical research is better described by a more flexible and heterogeneous view of normal science than Kuhn's paradigm. In normal periods of biophysical science paradigms are not single encompassing ideas but consist of many concepts and an abundance of methodological assumptions from physics, chemistry, and evolution. General hypotheses serve as paradigms, but they consist of parts that are continually changing: the importance of nucleic acids led for a while to the paradigmatic central dogma that "DNA makes RNA makes protein." And this hypothesis persisted in some form while contradictory assumptions that RNA can act as enzymes that in turn make DNA nibbled at the edges of the central dogma. The paradigmatic central dogma served only as the beginning of genetic research, not as a paradigm with complete explanatory powers. The multitude of hypotheses about restriction enzymes, postgenetic modifications, signaling pathways, membrane bound receptors, Ras and Myc pathways, and the myriad of subfields, each with its assumptions, chemical constituents, and developing methodologies make up the paradigm of today's biological research, which inches ahead on many fronts simultaneously. There is no one static paradigm guiding normal biological research, no one-dimensional line of movement, but fields of research activity in which whole populations of scientists and ideas move into slightly different grounds. The identification of "normal" science in biophysics research can be maintained only by broadening the concept of a paradigm to include the evolving methods and findings of biochemistry and cellular and evolutionary biology, guided by the axioms and reasoning of thermodynamics, evolution, and environmental interactions. In the vibrant, interactive period of "normal" biophysical science, experiments result in continually changing hypotheses and facts rely on the validity of these small contributing, changing paradigms, which are assumed but often questioned in the same experiment. Normal periods of biological science with their unceasing, inclusive curiosity include many qualities that Kuhn originally attributed to revolutionary science. Scientific hypotheses with differing degrees of experimental and theoretical support are the paradigms of normal biological science. Kuhn originally described normal science as a period of puzzle solving where questions were answered by applying paradigmatic insights. In that sense today's biophysics is normal science, and in my opinion, the more normal it is the better. Normal biological science owes its strengths to its ability to solve problems, in the course of which it has invented new hypotheses and designed ingenious experiments. Insofar as the physical questions being asked about bio-logical systems can be answered in the immediate future, I believe it will be through innovative but essentially normal science.

Kuhn was originally dismissive of normal science, describing it as puz-zle solving—obviously not as exciting as the revolutionary science illustrated by Einstein's novel conceptualizations of relativity, the photoelectric effect, and Brownian motion in one year. However, his subsequent higher opinion of normal science was shown in an exchange with the eminent philosopher Karl Popper on the question of how science is distinguished from non-science. What are the criteria that define astronomy as a science but not astrology—and chemistry rather than alchemy?

In a written version of his longstanding opinion, Popper[4] argued that the defi-nition of science depends upon its ability to formulate revolutionary hypotheses that can ultimately be falsified by experiment. For Popper science was distin-guished by its ability to disprove hypotheses; falsifiability distinguished science from non-science. For Popper new concepts created revolutions—concepts drove practice. My views are in sympathy with Kuhn's response,[5] the gist of which is that a "careful look at the scientific enterprise suggests that it is normal science, where Sir Karl's sort of testing does not occur, rather than extraordi-nary science which most clearly distinguishes science from other enterprises." In this exchange Kuhn had moved far from his early disparagement of normal science as mere "puzzle solving." By the time of his exchange with Popper he had come to see the modern technological world as the fruit of that same nor-mal science.

Our reevaluation of the period of normal science to include changing ideas requires that the nature of revolutionary science, as originally described by Kuhn and continued by Popper, must also be reevaluated to reflect existing practices in contemporary biophysical research. Kuhn's original version was that scientific revolutions were driven by free-floating concepts—derived, of course, from experimental data—but revolutions were caused abruptly by original concepts and scientific practice followed. However, it has been shown from historical examples by Steven Shapin, among others, that even in physics more continuous changes in scientific practice have led to widespread changes in science that, in retrospect, are called a scientific revolution. The opening sen-tence of his book *The Scientific Revolution*[6] summarizes this position: "There was no such thing as the Scientific Revolution and this is a book about it." Shapin describes how contributions from a group of scientists, wealthy ama-teurs, technically proficient machinists and gentlemen with a belief in honest testable results, created an advance in our understanding that, in time, installed the great explanatory powers of physics. He does not argue that conceptual advances were missing from seventeenth-century England but from historical evidence suggests a softening of the description of revolution based upon the sudden replacement of existing paradigms by a free-floating idea. This description of a more gradual evolution of a changing practice under the broad wings of a paradigm, resulting in a revolution, is, in my opinion, a more accurate description of the changes that take place in biophysics. Knowledge that DNA was involved in inheritance stimulated Watson and Crick to doggedly persist in physical studies of its molecular structure, which, as they note, showed a base-pairing whose significance for inheritance did not escape their notice. What followed from the experiments stimulated by the DNA research was the ongoing revolution of molecular genetics.

Popper's emphasis upon the importance of falsifiability assumes that free-floating ideas have the power to change scientific directions. This contrasts with Shapin's history, in which practice changes concepts so that revolutions are built gradually by changes in procedures that are simultaneously developing and creating new paradigms. Of course, both descriptions of the pace of revolutions have descriptive powers, but to the extent that revolutions in a field are initiated by novel concepts, the field is less stable. Advocates of large-scale revolutionary changes, such as are often envisaged for the new fields of genomics, systems biology, and Cognitive Neuroscience, contend that this is not a time for normal science. The claim, usually quite explicit, is that the strengths of modern physical science allow us to face questions about human activities and properties that previously could not be addressed by physical science. However, the danger posed by this kind of revolutionary science is that hypotheses will be accepted without the kind of testing that has given physical science its reliability. If a revolutionary proposal is believed before validation, it is quite possible that research will assume that these hypotheses have the reliability of physical science. In this event, untested *a priori* hypotheses could become the starting assumptions of biophysical experiments. Given the difficulties in disproving a hypothesis, the very belief that ideas can readily change a field can lead to a period when understanding is deduced from untested assumptions. In that event, deductive science, based upon unreliable hypotheses, will replace the reliable laws of chemistry and physics that have carefully been constructed from well-tested hypotheses.

THE REACH OF DEDUCTIVE REASONING

If proposals are assumed before they have been tested, then they form the basis of deductive science. Only when we realize that confidence in these assumptions has been misplaced, usually after time has shown their failings, do we realize that science has been done deductively, reasoning from a principle that turns out to be false. Biophysical research may be more likely than physical science to be deductive because its diversity allows unexamined assumptions to cross the many disciplinary boundaries and to be accepted as truths already established in other disciplines. For a Bell Labs physicist, unpaired electrons in DNA were unexpected and aroused excitement, but could be tested and dismissed summarily. In neuroscience, as we have seen, concepts about mental processes from psychology have gained traction in neuroimaging experiments in part because they come with the authority of another scientific field.

The need to distinguish between normal scientific research and deductive science was recognized early in the developments of nineteenth-century physiology. In a lecture given in the late nineteenth century, Hermann von Helmholtz protested against the introduction of untested hypotheses into biophysical research and showed that deductions from these assumptions, prevailing in the research of his day, were inhibiting discovery.[7] Trained as both a physicist and a physician, von Helmholtz is an excellent role model for modern biophysicists. As a leading researcher and a powerful figure in the German scientific community, he accepted the responsibility of explaining scientific advances to the layman. In his popular lectures and exhibits, which dealt with such topics as the wave nature of sound and how the inner ear recognized music by its harmonic contents, he frequently emphasized the importance of scientific and methodological advances by relating them to philosophical traditions.

In an address titled "On Thought in Medicine," presented to the Institute for the Education of Military Surgeons in 1877, von Helmholtz reflected upon the advances in medical science in the 35 years since he had been a student there.[7] Then, he recalled, medicine had been in ferment over "the fight between learned tradition and the new spirit of natural science." Subsequently, medicine had undergone a metamorphosis that provided "an instructive lesson on the true principles of scientific enquiry." Recognizing that the struggle for a new science could best be described in terms of natural philosophy, he went on to explain the "principles of scientific method" responsible for overturning the "learned tradition" of medicine that had prevailed in his student days:

> The fundamental error of that former time [was that] it pursued a false ideal of science in a one-sided and erroneous reverence for the deductive method… [and] in no other science have the consequences been so glaring, or have so hindered progress, as in medicine…. Earlier practitioners thought they could deduce, before they had settled their general principles by induction. They forgot that a deduction can have no more certainty than the principle from which it is deduced;… [their] essential and fundamental error [was] the false kind of logical conclusion… the conception

that it must be possible to build a complete system which would embrace all forms of disease, and their cure, upon any one…simple explanation.[8]

In von Helmholtz's lifetime, and to a great extent through his research, the deductive system was replaced in medical and physiological studies by modern physical experiments that led to the proposal and testing of hypotheses. Among the general principles that were taken as truths in his day, he was particularly critical of the powers assumed for the "vital force," whose claims to uncontested certitude discouraged experiments as unnecessary. Discredited practices such as therapeutic bloodletting had become medical panaceas, derived from physicians' belief in the four cardinal fluids—"representatives of the four classical elements, blood, phlegm, black and yellow gall"—that had earlier inhibited the characterization and treatment of specific diseases. Von Helmholtz went on to explain that the great laws established by physicists like Newton were based not on unquestioned universal truths, but rather on mathematical relationships that correlated existing observations and allowed them to be tested by further experimental results.

Deductive science can be identified as studies conducted and conclusions reached by assuming the validity of hypotheses that have not been validated by experimental tests. It is evident to us that maintaining the balance of the cardinal fluids is not a defining property of a healthy body. Freed from this universal "explanation" of disease, modern medicine has created a vast assortment of mechanisms, properties, and hypotheses that are more effective in treating disease than were treatments like bloodletting based upon the assumptions about cardinal fluids. We have replaced dependence upon the four cardinal fluids with the understanding developed from modern chemistry and biology. Instead of assuming that the body maintains these four fluids in balance, we assume its actions follow the laws of physics and chemistry, and biological research explores how these sciences exert their influence on bodily processes. However, the allure of rapid advances promised by free-floating ideas continues to draw researchers into deductive science.

NEW SCIENCE OR THE END OF SCIENCE

Deductive science today, as in von Helmholtz's time, is more common in the biological and medical sciences than in the physical sciences. The common backgrounds of physical and chemical studies place restraints on the flow of ideas between physical specialties, while the many disciplines contributing to the life sciences are a rich breeding ground for diverse conceptualizations and theories that can move across biomedical studies. The structures of these interdisciplinary activities are examined in the following chapters, where methods for integrating multidisciplinary insights are evaluated. The importance of understanding the nature of interdisciplinary studies is emphasized by the public notice such scientific directions are receiving. The difficulty of promising practical results from the support of basic research, although it can point to our modern world for support, has led to an apparent juggling of belief and disbelief and has raised concerns about the healthiness of science in our time.

For some this has raised the question of whether we are living through the "end of science." In his book of that title,[9] John Horgan, a perceptive science writer, interviewed prominent scientists about the nature of their science. He concluded that the empirical tests of hypotheses that characterized science in the past are no longer the only methods being advocated. Instead, large explanatory directions that are impossible to test are being proposed for the study of life and the world. Today's scientists, Horgan writes, "pursue science in a speculative, post empirical mode" that "resembles literary criticism in that it offers points of view, opinions, which are, at best, interesting, which provoke further comment. But it does not converge on the truth."[10] In his view, the neglect of testability has brought science into concordance with Harold Bloom's analysis of literature, in which all writers create "under the anxiety of influence" in efforts to reach beyond the great achievements of past writers.

In explaining the perceived need for new methodologies, Horgan observed that some scientists feel that the truly great scientific advances have already been made. In an effort to compete with those achievements, some new-style scientists have begun to promise more than established scientific methods can deliver. In one salient example of the replacement of traditional physical methods by deductive methods, Edward Witten, a highly respected theoretical physicist, told Horgan that the theory of superstrings was supported so strongly by its conceptual beauty and universality that it was as evident as "the sky is blue."[11] Other scientists interviewed by Horgan made similarly sweeping assertions, framing both questions and answers with absolute certainty. These modern proposals, of which superstrings are but one example, have the appearance of revolutionary hypotheses but, he suggests, include neither proven methods nor standards for testability.

The semipopular scientific literature abounds with proposals by eminent modern scientists to study systemic properties on the basis of novel *a priori* assumptions. We are familiar with the claims of particle theorists that universal truths of "what is" will be explained by an elusive "final theory."[12] In the same vein, particle experimentalists propose that everything will be explained by a "God particle"[13] and the answers will be found by building larger particle accelerators. The particular broad claim that I am contesting in these pages has been widely used to plan and interpret functional imaging experiments based on computational theories of mind. In these theories the mind is assumed to be a Turing machine that is "as general as any symbol-manipulating device can be."[14] Moreover, Fodor continues, "Turing machines are closed computational systems—the sole determinants of their commutations are the current machine state, the tape configurations and the program, the rest of the world being quite irrelevant." Since organisms are forever exchanging information with their environment, it is necessary that they be embedded in subsidiary systems "that are responsive to the flow of environmental events." To handle these inputs, Fodor notes that "faculty psychology is getting to be respectable again after centuries of hanging out with phrenologists and other dubious types."[15] He explains, "By faculty psychology I mean, roughly, that many fundamentally different kinds of psychological mechanisms must be postulated in order to explain the facts of mental life." The nature of these faculties, he continues, will be assumed to be modular. In this model, Fodor continues, "overt, observable behavior is an interaction effect par excellence."[15] Fodor recognizes that this model of mind is reviving "Descartes' doctrine of innate ideas . . . a theory about how the mind is (initially, intrinsically, genetically) structured into psychological faculties."[16] I will return to this model of mind in the following pages, but to start I assert that it has been responsible for degrading neuroimaging experiments into the deductivism that has vitiated the field and that the empirical, inductive approach to brain studies that I am endorsing stands in opposition to this model in every way examined. In contrast to these assumptions about intrinsic properties of brain and mind, I shall be presenting evidence obtained by the experimental studies characteristic of normal science that emphasizes the initially homogeneous and undifferentiated state of mind that is developed in the individual by experience.

Horgan extended his investigatory interviews to leaders of brain science, and his subsequent volume[17] examines mind-related science. Horgan was able to interview a full cast of eminent brain scientists, providing a detailed, informative view of the enthusiasms, opinions, and results of neuroscience at the end of the last millennium. Horgan not only presented their views but also came to conclusions about the state and promise of neuroscience. In contrast to his earlier broader review of science, he felt that neuroscience will not come to an end because people will never tire of trying to understand themselves and their minds and feelings. But given the unconvincing progress he found in neuroscience, he concluded that "Given their poor record to date I fear that neuroscience . . . and other fields addressing the mind might be bumping up against fundamental limits of science."[18] Horgan found that many of the neuroscientists claim to have spanned the "Explanatory Gap," which is the "inability of physiological theories to account for psychological phenomena." Or, as he concluded in admiration of the detailed research in the field: "mind-scientists excel at taking the brain apart, but they have no idea how to put it back together again."[19] The next chapter traces the philosophical origins of these diametrically opposed views of mind and begins to assemble the philosophical, historical, and experimental support for a view of mind that incorporates the Pragmatist's flexibility into an empirical study of behavior and avoids the uncertainties of psychological assumptions.

NOTES

1. Barnett, L., Brenner, S., Crick, F. H. C., Shulman, R. G., & Watts-Tobin R. (1967) Phase-shift and other mutants in the first part of the rIIB cistron of bacteriophage T4. *Philosophical Transactions of the Royal Society Part B,* 252:487.
2. Those of us who mourn the breakup of the Bell System and the consequent loss of Bell Telephone Laboratories as a once-great national treasure are comforted by the way in which the principles of Bell Labs' research philosophy have been revived in the corridors of power. Steven Chu, a Bell Labs alumnus who is now Secretary of Energy, has incorporated the essence of the labs' trust in individual scientists into the Department of Energy's plans to create original directions for energy research.
3. Kuhn, T. S. (1962). *The structure of scientific revolutions.* Chicago: University of Chicago Press.
4. Popper, K. (1998). Science: Conjectures and refutations. In M. Curd & J. A. Cover (Eds.), *Philosophy of science: The central issues* (pp. 3–10). New York & London: W.W. Norton & Company.
5. Kuhn, T. S. (1998). Logic of discovery or psychology of research. In M. Curd & J. A. Cover (Eds.), *Philosophy of science: The central issues* (pp. 11–19). New York & London: W.W. Norton & Company.
6. Shapin, S. (1996). *The scientific revolution* (p. 1). Chicago & London: University of Chicago Press.
7. von Helmholtz, H. (1877). "On Thought in Medicine," an address delivered on August 2, 1877. In D. Cahan (Ed.), *Science and culture: Popular and philosophical essays* (p. 309). Chicago & London: University of Chicago Press.
8. Ibid. (pp. 311–315).
9. Horgan, J. (1996). *The end of science.* Reading, MA: Helix Books, Addison-Wesley Publishing Co.
10. Ibid. (p. 7).
11. Ibid. (p. 60).
12. Weinberg, S. (1994). *Dreams of a final theory.* New York: Vintage Books, A Division of Random House.
13. Lederman, L., & Teresi, D. (1993). *The God particle: If the universe is the answer, what is the question?* New York: Dell.
14. Fodor, J. (1983). *The modularity of mind* (p. 39). Cambridge, MA, & London: MIT Press.
15. Ibid. (p. 1).

16. Ibid. (p. 3).
17. Horgan, J. (1999). *The undiscovered mind: How the human brain defies replication, medication and explanation.* New York: Touchstone.
18. Ibid. (p. 10).
19. Ibid. (p. 23).

3

A Philosophical Background

What use can philosophy be to a physical scientist who is studying brain activities in the hope that reliable physical methods will illuminate mental functions? Why should we turn to philosophy, a notoriously difficult subject that requires understanding highly developed technical terms, to clarify things that seem very clear to experimentalists? My answer is that we cannot avoid basing our scientific work on philosophical choices; the question is whether we want to make philosophical decisions knowledgeably or without intending to do so. At every step of a functional imaging experiment choices are made about the nature of mental processes that are so commonly accepted in our culture that they do not appear to have been influenced by a philosophical position but rather seem "obvious." However, even the seemingly straightforward decision to study brain function by physical methods places us squarely in one camp of a philosophical controversy that goes back at least as far as Descartes.

Both the modern physical sciences and their philosophical underpinnings trace their origins to a turning point in the early seventeenth century. The so-called Scientific Revolution was characterized by hopes for understanding nature, often supported by novel methodologies, as well as by a struggle against worldviews that, as late as Newton's day, rested on theological canons and authority. Although the founders of modern physics were replacing the existing understanding of the material world, their enquiries into the soul and mind were limited by an orthodoxy about mental function that only recently is being questioned by modern brain science. To identify views that may have outlasted their utility, it is helpful to consider how science in the seventeenth century made the transition from the assumptions of scholasticism to the present model of empirical science, with its inductive-hypothetical methodology. This transition is most conspicuous in the life of Galileo Galilei.[1]

GALILEO AND THE POWERS OF OBSERVATION

Galileo was born in 1564 in Pisa to an impoverished Florentine family; his father was a competent mathematician and an able musician and a member of the musical circle that created the secular music of madrigals and eventually the first operas. At an early age, Galileo was appointed to a post at Pisa, where his mathematical training, coupled with a belief in his own powers of observation, brought him to positions that differed from the prevailing orthodoxy. In 1592 he moved to Padua, where he flourished under the more permissive rule of Venice. There he did his important physical research on moving bodies until 1610, when his move to Florence placed him under the protection of the Medici and simultaneously the telescope made astronomical observations possible. Galileo's long (1564–1642) and productive life makes any summary impossible, but it is possible to discern themes in his studies that are relevant for our investigations of neuroscience.

THE CREATION OF PHYSICS

In Pisa Galileo is known to have started studies of the new science concerned with the acceleration of falling bodies, the constancy of the pendulum, and the parabolic path of projectiles. His experimental studies on falling bodies showed, in one of his rare well-documented actual experiments, that objects do not fall with a velocity proportional to their weight. His reliance on observation allowed him to determine orderly properties of substances, which, coupled with his mathematical training, he subsequently systematized into mathematical laws of motion, thereby creating modern physics. These findings, although widely known, were not published as a systematic science until 1638. His criticisms of the laws of moving bodies, accepted since Aristotle, were there presented as mathematical laws of motion. Although Galileo did not extend mathematical physics to the motion of heavenly bodies (this great synthesis of universal gravitation was left to Newton), his assertion of the universality of physical laws and his formulation of the laws of bodies accelerating under the force of gravity laid the foundation for classical physics. In the early stage of his physical studies, before enough regularity had been described to support mathematical descriptions, Galileo faced disorganized experimental and conceptual results, a combination of authoritarian views, recent theories, and scattered observations that led him to propose a scientific method, different from the mathematical laws of motion he subsequently developed. In writing about sunspots in 1613 Galileo proposed to avoid the search for the essence of things, which was characteristic of the comprehensive descriptions offered by Aristotelian science:

Either we want, by theorizing, to try to penetrate the true and intrinsic essence of natural substances, or we want to limit ourselves to gain information about some of their properties. As for trying to penetrate the essence, I regard it as an undertaking and a job no less impossible and useless for the case of nearby elementary substances than for the case of heavenly and very remote substances. I feel equally ignorant of about the substance of the earth and the moon, or terrestrial clouds and of sunspots.[2]

It is of no little interest for neuroscience, a rather new subject, that in the early studies of motion Galileo was not enthusiastic about mathematical laws that provided necessary and sufficient explanations of motion—they were to come later. His interest in the empirical properties of natural substances shows what can be expected in the early phases of a field. His emphasis on the need to understand the observable properties of matter was to lay the foundation for the inductive-empirical tradition of quantitative science, which emphasizes the push–pull relationship between induction and empirical testing.

THE COPERNICAN SOLAR SYSTEM

The studies that formed the foundation of modern physics continued until the end of Galileo's time in Padua in 1609, when he turned his attention to the heavenly bodies. Reports of the telescope invented in Holland stimulated Galileo to design and build telescopes of increasing power and optical quality.

From his original astronomical observations of the moons of Jupiter, of the shadows on Earth's moon, and of the erratic motion of sunspots moving across the face of the sun, Galileo argued that the heavens were not perfect Earth-centered spheres and that the same laws could describe heavenly and earthly motions. These contradictions of the Aristotelian premise of perfect circular motions of celestial bodies supported his lifelong goal of unifying earthly and celestial motions. Our appreciation of Galileo's insight is heightened by our awareness of the fragility of his information. Galileo was not reasoning logically, but rather inferring boldly, from similarities he observed between the earthly and celestial bodies, that they would broadly follow the same laws. His criticism of the Aristotelian circular motion, the Church's explanation of the motion of heavenly bodies, left the Copernican model as the most likely alternative, supported by the simpler description it offered. Galileo struggled to find experimental distinctions between the two models, at one time relying on theories about the tides that were based on mistaken data. The most convincing reason came from the motion of sunspots, which as they moved across the surface of the sun could be more simply explained by a Copernican model in which the Earth moved around the sun than by an Earth-centered view.

Journeying to Rome in 1616, he had been forced to promise not to "hold, teach or defend" the forbidden doctrine. However, his continuing support for Copernicus resulted in his condemnation for heresy in 1634, and he remained under house arrest until his death 8 years later. His willingness to stand by his scientific observations and their interpretation even when this placed him in peril is the paradigmatic historical example of the powers of science to defend philosophical positions.

HUMAN STUDIES

The wide range of Galileo's research compelled him to ask what properties of matter qualified it for study and what other phenomena were best excluded. Galileo had limited expectations as to what could be found from the study of humans. His knowledge of optics, in particular, led him to develop a sophisticated position on the relationship between the observer and the phenomenon. He described the difference between the observer's senses and the kinetics of matter in a statement that limited physical studies to material bodies:

I simultaneously feel the necessity of conceiving that it [matter] has boundaries and is of some shape or other; that relatively to others it is great or small; that it is in this or that place, in this or that time; that it is in motion or at rest.... I am inclined to think that these tastes, smells, colors etc. with regard to the object in which they appear to reside, are nothing more than mere names, and exist only in the sensitive body; in so much that when the living creature is removed, all these qualities are carried off and annihilated; although we have imposed our particular names upon them...and would fain persuade ourselves that they truly and in fact exist.[3]

The distinction between matter, which exists in place, time, and space and which can be measured against an objective scale, and our *impression* of such matter, which resides in ourselves and is a property of our perception, would come to mark the fundamental boundary of physical science. In time, perceptions and the body's reaction to them would be developed into psychology and physiology. By confining itself to inorganic material substances, early physics asserted both its objectivity and the freedom to study the forces and laws that described the motion and attraction of material bodies. At least as important, however, is Galileo's contribution in advising us what *not* to study. By carefully defining what could be studied (the motion of matter) and what could not (its subjective taste, smell, or color), he formulated a physics whose findings have come to epitomize scientific validity. The world is divided into those things that are amenable to study reliably with his inductive method (at a given historical moment) and those that are not. For Galileo, the motion of planets could be studied with the telescopes of his day, while the physiology of vision could not. (Arguably, the subjective character of vision remains elusive to this day.) This was a reasonable scientific position because, for example, no effort on his part could have unraveled the process by which light causes a depolarization of the retina that travels to the occipital cortex via the optic nerve; the biological advances leading to those insights lay in the distant future. Over time, however, the very physical sciences that Galileo helped to invent, among them neuroscience, began to chip away at the foundation of what we might call Galilean dualism.

DESCARTES' DUALISM

In the differences between the Cartesian world and the creation of physics by Galileo and Newton we can distinguish the overlapping claims of deductive and empirical science that we are trying to disentangle in modern biophysics.

Born in France in 1596, Descartes was educated by Jesuits and ultimately settled in Holland, where his experience as an émigré shaped his view of the world.[4] In contrast to Galileo's investigations in the freer spirit of the Italian Renaissance, Descartes saw man's life in the state of nature as solitary, with an almost churlish combativeness, similar to the views of his contemporary (and correspondent) Thomas Hobbes.[5] During his own short life (he died in Sweden in 1650), Descartes published treatises that revolutionized mathematics, science, and philosophy. The breathtaking scope of Descartes' investigations dooms any attempt to fit them into a simple pattern. We will nevertheless attempt to touch on a few elements that play important roles in modern neuroscience.

Taking precautions from Galileo's conflict with the Church, Descartes published a heavily abridged and self-censored autobiographical account of his philosophical system in 1635.[5] Like Galileo, he dismissed the Aristotelian philosophy that had been incorporated into the theology of his day. Also like Galileo, he was gravely concerned with the question of what topics were appropriate for study with the available investigative tools. However, Descartes' skepticism led him to very different conclusions. Rejecting empirical knowledge as not dependable, he concluded that observation of nature was not a suitable basis for the certainty he sought. Scholarship of the time was not built upon reproducible, quantitative observations; more often than not, it was intended either to illustrate Aristotle's descriptions of the natural world or to explain anomalies, such as the two-headed snakes in today's sensational press. In an attempt to find the "Method of Rightly Conducting the Reason and Seeking for

Truth in the Sciences,"[6] Descartes resolved to ignore empirical knowledge and to accept nothing that was not presented to his mind so clearly and distinctly that it could not be doubted.

While still in his twenties, Descartes had invented modern analytical geometry by fusing geometry and algebra. The combination of these two abstract, non-empirical fields provided novel solutions to practical, real-world material problems, including many that had puzzled the ancient Greeks, such as how to double the volume of a cube. Inspired by his successes with analytical geometry, Descartes hoped to explain corporeal phenomena by making deductions from analogous intuitive concepts. These *a priori* assumptions were to be "clear and distinct" and, above all, incontrovertible. Unlike empirical studies that could be contaminated by observer errors, deductions from intuition would retain their absolute validity. Finding in his mind a certitude that existed nowhere else, Descartes asserted that "I think, therefore I am,"[6] stating an absolute truth, completely certain. (He expressed confidence in his new deductive method on the same page of the great treatise that describes his procedure for breaking the whole down into parts, an approach that is regarded as a cornerstone of modern empirical science.) Certainty was to be found in his mind, which he fused with the religious concept of soul (*âme*); for, as Descartes said, "the soul by which I am what I am."[7] Both concepts were considered intuitively obvious.

Descartes' method was to deduce logical conclusions from the intuitively certain knowledge (or statement) that he did think. From the assumption that he was capable of thought, he deduced that he existed, and from this he went on to conclude that the mind had an immaterial nature that differed starkly from what his assumptions and findings, some quite similar to Galileo's, revealed about corporeal matter. Descartes' certitude concerning the existence of mind contrasted with his skepticism about the vagaries and doubts of observation. Mind, in the worldview of Cartesian dualism, is something different from matter. It may interact with the physical world but it is not of it, nor can its truths be contradicted by observation. Such views are shocking (and sometimes risible) to modern audiences surrounded by evidence of the concrete advances to be achieved by trusting observations of material bodies. We will see below how Descartes' certainties continue to tilt neuroscience away from the empiricism I am advocating. But first it merits mentioning that he was far less dogmatic in his material studies than were his followers. Indeed, Descartes was a tireless and innovative experimental scientist. His research ranged over all matter, animate and inanimate, and provided critical support to the incipient sciences of physiology and physics. In one of his many experiments, he calculated how the different refraction of light in air and water explained the observed angular bend of primary and secondary rainbows.[8] In the course of his investigations he developed hypotheses, retaining those that explained observations and occasionally modifying or discarding them in response to criticism. This proponent of a deductive science based upon untested assumptions was at the same time an early practitioner of inductive-hypothetical science—an inconsistency from the modern perspective, but one that was probably inevitable during the revolutionary transition from scholastic definitions to modern scientific methodology.[9] The tensions in Descartes' science between questionable *a priori* assumptions and empirically testable hypotheses were resolved by others, most notably Galileo and Newton. Yet half a century later Cartesian essentialists still faulted Newton for failing to provide an *a priori* explanation of gravitational force. For these critics, the laws of gravity were useful generalizations of Kepler's observations but unimportant compared to what Newton had not supplied—namely, their derivation from uncontestable *a priori* understanding of the force of gravity. In these criticisms we see an early conflict in physical science between the deductive and inductive-empirical approaches that continue to this day to animate neuroscience.

DESCARTES' MIND IS THE PROBLEM

Philosophical treatment of mind can be considered as having started with Descartes' arguments for the dualism of mind and matter, of the immaterial and the material, as well as their incommensurability. To modern sensibilities, it is somewhat surprising that for Descartes the mind was known with absolute certainty while the material world was only insecurely perceived, beset as it was by dreams, hallucinations, and reports that emphasized unusual phenomena. This view of mind, in which its properties were intuitively known to the individual by unmediated, direct self-knowledge, persists to this day. It is expressed in the attitude that we know who we are and what we intend; in our confidence in the everyday impressions of our own minds; and in the common assumption that the same sorts of things are true of other people's minds. Philosophy and psychology have taken up Descartes' challenge of describing how mind represented the external, material world; the result of these centuries of philosophical explorations is that philosophical considerations of the meaning of mind now pervade our culture.

Many philosophers have followed Descartes by assuming the existence of a mind and to study it have followed either "materialism" or "dualism."[10] Dualism and materialism both assume that mental processes are valid descriptions of the world and differ only by their optimism about the possibility of explaining these descriptions by material activities such as brain functions. In the materialistic view, all mental activities can ultimately be explained by physical mechanisms of the brain. Our emotions, thoughts, and intents are considered by materialists to be explainable by the activities of the brain with varying degrees of the completeness characteristic of physical science. For materialists, uncertainties about the nature of mind are insignificant compared to the challenge of mapping its properties onto brain processes.

Dualists, on the other hand, also follow Descartes in distinguishing between mental activities and material events. Although they often allow for the brain to be involved in the mechanisms responsible for the mental, dualists nonetheless view mental processes as a nonphysical element of reality, but assume they cannot be explained by material mechanisms such as brain activities. Thomas Nagel's dualism of mental and scientific understanding presents an example of the dualist position. Nagel claims an irreconcilable brain/mind dualism and considers this relationship between the objective brain and the subjective mind to be the central question of philosophy. He does not seek to unify them into a single worldview, warning that attempts to unify personal conceptions of life and the world with objective science lead to philosophical mistakes and false reductions.[11] Instead, he proposes "to juxtapose the internal and external or subjective and objective views at full strength, in order to achieve unification when it is possible and to recognize clearly when it is not."[12] Nagel is intent upon preserving the subjective, personal nature of human life, its judgments, sensations, and values, and resists the claim that such thoughts and feelings can be expressed in objective physical terms since he claims that the language of physics is "too impoverished" to describe them. Nagel states the problem so as to make integration difficult and apparently impossible. His popular description of the difficulties that hinder our understanding in an essay on the mind of a bat emphasizes the inconceivable remoteness of the insoluble questions raised by the problem he has created.[12]

Nagel, like many other philosophers, proposes to define what is normative for brain studies, what scientists should and should not do. However, as a neuroscientist I am not convinced that philosophers can offer a more valid description of the epistemological limitations of neuroscience than can be found in the scientific history of the subject. Nagel's claim of an irreconcilable dualism differs sharply from the goals for neuroscience proposed in this book, which aim to clarify connections between brain activities and the behavioral functions they serve.

As we leave Descartes (and his intellectual inheritors) for the moment, it is important to review the strong influences that his ideas have had on both scientific method and the philosophy of mind. He emphasized the importance and the very existence of mind while at the same time defining it so as to be inaccessible to scientific knowledge. This posed a challenge to the powers of science, and as the complexity of the problem grew by accumulated philosophical enquiries, it became the Gordian knot preventing scientific study of human behavior by interjecting the need to understand the properties of mind presumed to underlie that behavior. We have already seen the important contributions that Pragmatism has made to this traditional philosophical concern, to cutting this knot, by proposing that descriptions of mental processes are but words and that by focusing on the meaning of words like "beauty," "truth," or "working memory," philosophers (and scientists) are introducing contingent subjective conceptualities into the study of the objective reality they are trying to describe.

PRAGMATISM AND THE CONTINGENCY OF THOUGHT

The realization that our understanding is constructed by humans plays a central role in the Pragmatist reformulation of the connection between brain activities and mental processes. The assumptions about essential properties of mind developed by traditional philosophers, following Descartes, and taken for granted in everyday discourse have been countered by the philosophy of Pragmatism developed by William James, John Dewey, Ludwig Wittgenstein, and Richard Rorty. Pragmatism opposes the traditional philosophical ideas about the meaningfulness of descriptions of mental processes that have been accepted and reinforced by the growing collectivism of biological science. Pragmatist planning and interpretation of experiments can relate brain activities to behavior experimentally instead of following the traditional philosophical and societal assumptions, which lead into the uncertainties of mental processes. The Pragmatist restatement of philosophy eliminates many of the traditional arguments formulated by everyday language. A fundamental difference with everyday language can be found in the Pragmatists' usage of "mind."[13] In contrast to the confidence with which traditional Western philosophers, represented above by Thomas Nagel, propose that they understand mind, or its stand-ins of long-term memory or attention, Pragmatists propose that the concept of mind, while extremely useful in many aspects of everyday life, is really a construct that humans have created because it helps us deal with the world. In this formulation the concept of mind is not to be found in the world, nor is it a representation of something in the world; rather, it is a contingent term whose value depends upon the actions it leads to in a particular time, person, and place. There is no objective definition of mind that can be identified with a specific brain process and location, since all definitions depend upon its user and its context. The possibility of locating such concepts in the brain, even for the limited goal of being necessary for the person's behavior, is denied by the Pragmatist's understanding that such concepts do not exist outside of their particular usages. Assuming the validity of such "everyday" concepts has created the difficulties in neuroscience experiments revealed in the working memory experiments described in the first chapter. Philosophers in the Pragmatist camp have supported this innate skepticism by expressing a criticism of these concepts and the general intellectual processes that give them such apparent solidity.

In the aftermath of World War I, Ludwig Wittgenstein, who had been trained as an engineer, constructed his philosophy upon advances in logic and questioned any attempt to formulate the nature of abstract qualities in language. He was troubled by the difficulty of defining not just abstractions like "beauty" and "truth" but also the words that we use to name everyday objects with the rigor required of mathematical logic. In his view, the "craving for generality" arises from the mistaken idea that properties we use to describe phenomena, such as beauty and truth, are in fact ingredients; that, as he put it, beauty is an "ingredient of all beautiful things as alcohol is of beer and wine."[14] He felt that the conviction that generalizations are "scientific," since they reduce natural phenomena to a small number of general laws, shows contempt for the specific and thus impedes knowledge. In one of many examples, Wittgenstein noted how mathematical proofs about a limited set of cardinal numbers were treated contemptuously by mathematicians because they could not be proven to be universally true.[15]

Wittgenstein's achievement was not to bemoan the inadequacy of generalizations but to use symbolic logic to show what could be represented in language—and, more important, what could not. He argued that the range of what language could say with certainty was limited to an area roughly coincident with mathematics. Why, Wittgenstein asked, do philosophers have trouble defining chairs or tables, when every 6-year-old knows how to use these words? We teach a child the meaning of these words, he continued, not by abstract definitions but by example. To define chair, we point to this chair and then to that chair, and soon the child knows what the word means. Then we test him, and if he points to his hat or to the ceiling when asked to point to a chair, we offer him more examples until finally he gets the idea. In using the word "chair," the child is not bewildered when we point to a throne or a doll's house miniature chair or a three-legged chair and ask if they are chairs. "Well," he might respond, "they are chairs, sort of." Any attempt to formulate a definition of chair that applies equally well to all chairs while excluding all non-chairs is doomed and is of no interest to us or to the child we are teaching. Such exercises are simply pointless, Wittgenstein argued, and when philosophers struggle to find the rules of that game, it merely shows them to be less intelligent than a 6-year-old.

In summarizing this conclusion in the ominous final words of the only book he published during his lifetime, Wittgenstein wrote, "Whereof one cannot speak, thereof one must be silent."[14] Thus did he attack all forms of rational systems, particularly theories of ethics and aesthetics that would deduce human values by reasoning from general principles that were simply far too imprecise to be useful. Wittgenstein did not claim that morality was contrary to reason, "merely that its foundations lay elsewhere." So, in contradistinction to the sweeping claims made for reason, Wittgenstein located "the basis of morality in 'right feelings' rather than in `valid Reasons.'"[15]

Those of us who follow Wittgenstein accept that current science does not have the conceptual or material tools to provide an abstract, objective definition of mind, any more than we can rigorously define a chair. We do not believe that logic and reason alone can provide physically reliable insight into subjective experience. In the realm of the personal, nothing can be assumed with the assurance associated with mathematics, or even the empirical laws of classical physics. No generalizations from the personal, from common sense, from psychology, from the social sciences, from popular culture, or from everyday usage can be taken as a starting point from which reliable neuroscientific truths can be deduced.

Once we accept that generalizations of common objects cannot be defined with the degree of accuracy found in mathematics, it follows that less familiar entities, such as "working memory" and "attention," cannot be redefined in objective material terms by the images obtained from fMRI experiments. Like the words "chair" and "table," such generalizations are of considerable use in everyday speech, but in the physical sciences, which demand rigor in hypothesis testing, they set neuroscientists off on a futile chase, trying to ensnare a will-o'-the-wisp. To use Wittgenstein's example: when the child was limiting his scope of the word "chair" to demonstrable evidence-based usage, it was a valuable parallel. In the same way, building up careful experimental data will, I believe, get us "somewhere" useful in understanding the brain and its more complex functions. But the way there is not to be achieved by pursuing generalizations.

RICHARD RORTY AND PRAGMATISM

Richard Rorty's philosophy of Pragmatism provides another valuable perspective for disentangling psychological assumptions from neuroscientific measurements. Of the several origins of Pragmatism, Rorty paid particular attention to Wittgenstein's criticism of generalizations, and his conclusions—sometimes interpreted as a radical skepticism that can even be seen as nihilistic—are actually quite modest in reminding us about what we can "know." Rorty is a strong proponent of the view that philosophers like "great scientists invent descriptions of the world which are useful for purposes of predicting and controlling what happens, just as poets and political thinkers invent other descriptions of it for other purposes."[16] The world, he emphasizes, is concrete and not of our creation. Cause and effect operate independently of human mental activity. In contrast, all that can be understood by humans are the subjective descriptions of phenomena. Rorty's claim is that "where there are no sentences, there is no truth."[17] And sentences are human creations.

Contingency is central to Rorty's philosophy, since any description created to understand the world depends upon language and is determined by an individual's history and perspective. Language, metaphor, science, and imagination can all create understanding, Rorty proposes, but such understanding is necessarily contingent. We do not find scientific laws, he asserts; we create them. We do not find philosophical problems; we formulate them. Thus scientific discovery depends upon personal choice in a manner similar to all other creative acts. Where science differs, in Rorty's view, and differs in a way that really matters, is that its well-established methods of experimentation and reasoning have in many cases provided a high degree of validation of great usefulness, thereby reducing the degree of contingency.

In discussing the "causal character of mental concepts," Rorty writes that all our disciplines "are tools for coping with the world." For Pragmatists, people "are equally in touch with reality when they describe a hunk of space-time in atomic, molecular, cellular, physiological, behavioral, intentional, political or religious terms."[18] Hence there can be no philosophical interest in replacing one description with another purely for the sake of "conceptual clarity," because "Wittgenstein has taught us that clarity is a matter of ease and fruitfulness of use, not of translation into a preferred vocabulary." Rorty notes that between a small Phillips-head screwdriver and a large crescent wrench there are all sorts of similarities and differences, but none have ontological or epistemological significance. Nor can such invidious distinctions be made between, say, physics and literary criticism, although of course their usefulness will vary considerably with the occasion. Pragmatists evaluate efforts to relate any given discipline to another in terms of the utility of establishing such a relationship. In other words, the value of interdisciplinary studies is to be judged by the usefulness of the understandings they produce. This is important to the historical arc of scientific epistemology that I am tracing because it proposes that a concept borrowed from psychology or economics and brought into neuroscientific experimentation is not a "valid" basis for scientific experimentation, although it may be very useful in doing research in psychology or economics (or in daily life, for that matter). It is a tool that is valuable—or not—contingent upon its use.

By Rorty's standards, there is little reason not to pursue interdisciplinary studies in the unsettled brain/mind field; the issue is how such studies are to be conducted. Researchers must respect the varying degrees of reliability associated with different disciplines. In view of Wittgenstein's critique of generalizations, any assumptions about mind, including attempts to break it into components such as "working memory," must be avoided as mere philosophical word games, and are to be used only if they are useful rather than as insights that must be explained scientifically. Too often biophysical researchers feel driven to make certain assumptions about the nature of mental processes at the outset of their studies, rather than waiting until they have made substantial progress toward understanding the role these mental processes have been claimed to fulfill.

The method of scientific induction and testing that has evolved since Galileo is widely accepted in biophysics and neuroscience. The hypothetical-inductive approach, based on physical laws transplanted from the inanimate world, has proven itself both revealing and helpful. Scientific studies owe their strengths to their dependence upon well-understood physical methods that are the most reliable understanding we have at this time. And this is so despite the fact that the laws of classical mechanics, as codified in thermodynamics, are contingent human creations that can be overturned, just as other findings of classical mechanics have been qualified by relativity and quantum mechanics.

In a formal sense, the physical methods that I am proposing as the most reliable approach to understanding the brain are no different from the *a priori* assumptions of truth that I have criticized as unreliable. The crucial distinction is that the usefulness of the hypotheses and laws of physics has been tested and supported by centuries of scientific research. The same cannot be said of the qualities of mind that were assumed by Descartes, that have been delineated by subsequent philosophers, and that serve as the basis of many fMRI experiments.

THE SLIPPERY SLOPE

Does following pragmatism lead to a skepticism toward the value of science as a discipline, since some read Rorty as saying that science—like the world created by the poet—is merely a construct? Rorty has described these different degrees of certitude as falling on a spectrum with the end of great certainty held by physics and its allied disciplines.[19] However, lumping science with other disciplines as human efforts to understand the world may offend scientists, who often hold a view implicitly, and sometimes quite explicitly, that science discovers facts and truths that are not contingent but have absoluteness. The admiration of science by scientists and non-scientists alike is often based on the opinion that science is in possession of absolute truths—not of contingent hypotheses that have proven their worth by having survived tests. To the extent that those absolutist views of science are held, a scientist who advocates Pragmatism, with its disclaimer of unquestioned truths, is perceived as a heretic. Absolute truths can be abandoned, but the fear is aroused that once science is not qualitatively different from non-science, one is on a slippery slope of relativism, where all positions are equally valid—where once again alchemy competes with chemistry and astrology is the equal of astronomy. However, what I'm arguing is that even without absolute certainty about nature, science still provides the best insights and the most useful information that describes (and allows us to utilize) the material world. This is relevant to the story of this book because it is important to remember—as scientists—that we are always working within a set of philosophical assumptions about what we can know. Those who are pursuing their research under the assumption that *a priori* views of the mind (of the investigator) are able to assert the meaning of an abstract concept in a reliable way are following the deductive school of Descartes where some concepts are taken as true beyond the need for validation. Those who do not are by no means resigned to "all knowledge being slippery and contingent" (as extreme relativists would believe). They instead can hold on to (and celebrate) the pragmatic approach to testing knowledge by its utility. They too conduct research within a philosophical framework— one that neither over-claims the certainty of a scientific truth claim nor devalues the very real and very practical knowledge and insight into nature gained, tested, and utilized through inductive research.

FROM WITTGENSTEIN TO BENNETT AND HACKER

As long ago as 1934, Wittgenstein anticipated the perplexing issues raised by today's fMRI experiments in a prescient analysis of the possibility of brain imaging. When we speak of thinking as being located in the brain, he said, we are unconsciously drawing an analogy to such physical activities as writing and talking, which are clearly located in the hand or voice. But, he asked, "in what sense can the physiological processes be said to correspond to thoughts, and in what sense can we be said to get the thoughts from the observation of the brain?" Wittgenstein[20] envisioned an experimenter (who is also the subject of the experiment) being able to observe localized brain regions responding while in the process of thought. The subject-experimenter is looking for a correlation between thought and brain activity. "Both of these phenomena," Wittgenstein wrote, "could correctly be called 'experiences of thought,' and the question 'where is the thought itself?' had better, in order to prevent confusion, be rejected as nonsensical."

Maxwell Bennett and Peter Hacker,[21] expanding upon Wittgenstein's argument, take the metaphysical position that to talk about localizing a thought in the brain is nonsensical. They analyzed the work of cognitive neuroscientists and philosophers in discussing the mind–body problem in these terms. Their broad criticism of Cognitive Neuroscience is that it remains committed to flawed Cartesian views leading to conceptual confusions, in which psychological attributes (commonly considered identical with the mind) are ascribed to the brain. Cognitive Neuroscientists, they say, accept Descartes' account of mind and body and propose that it can be resolved by simply mapping the concepts of mind onto the brain. They show how in cognitive studies the psychological properties formerly assigned to mind are assumed to have been transferred to the brain, where—since the brain is material—they can presumably be studied scientifically. Hence the elusive personal properties of thought and belief, formerly assigned to mind, are now claimed by cognitive neuroscientists to be open to scientific understanding.

Bennett and Hacker claim that this transfer is conceptually wrong in that "it ascribes to the brain attributes that it makes sense only to ascribe to the animal as a whole."[22] This "mereological fallacy," wherein a property of the whole is assigned to a part, recalls, they say, Cartesian attribution of the existence of the self to the thinking mind. Bennett and Hacker claim that "it is not the brain that is conscious or unconsciousness, but the person whose brain it is. It is not the lecturer's brain but the lecturer, who becomes and is conscious of the ticking of the clock."[23] Bennett and Hacker's analysis leads to several fundamental clarifications about the methods for studying brain function. First, they reach the conclusion that the brain does not perform any of the mental functions postulated for it—it does not do memory or make decisions—but an active, healthy brain is necessary for the person to remember or to decide.

Second, the centrality of brain function necessary for behavior allows me to relate two observables and to bypass problems that have been created by the contingency of concepts of mental activity. The relationships to be understood are not between brain activity and mental concepts but between the necessary supports that brain activity offers and the person's behavior. The empirical question for functional imaging becomes not where mental activities are localized in the brain, but whether it is possible to identify brain activities that are necessary for the human to perform observable behavior.

Third, although brain activities are necessary for the person's performance or behavior, they do not cause the behavior: they are not both necessary and sufficient to cause or explain the person's behavior. The role that brain activity plays in supporting the person's behavior will be discussed in the next chapter, but it has already been indicated that brain studies can identify mechanisms that contribute to behavior. Their work, thus, gives us tools for being optimistic about the prospects for judicious neuroscience to make progress in eventually throwing light on some of the brain's more complex functions.

TRANSITION TO HISTORY

Philosophical analysis of neuroscience programs can provide valuable insight into their underlying assumptions and methods. It can relate practical decisions in the design of experiments to broader views of the nature assumed for mind or to the goals of a particular method. But such analyses do not in themselves establish scientific validity and usefulness, which depend on scientific insights and the present state of our knowledge. Only scientists can decide whether an assumption about the brain, even one that minimizes its subjective roots, provides a useful starting point for physical studies.

In the early seventeenth century scientists identified a limited world of inorganic phenomena that were the proper subject for physical study; at the same time, they took the useful step of reflecting upon their methods and articulating how their research depends upon *what they believe we can know and how they propose to know it.* Since then the boundaries of fields appropriate to observation and analysis have been continually enlarged to include life processes. The big leaps forward of the nineteenth-century physiologists illustrate a movement that continues to this day. Chemical and physical processes that Galileo and Descartes had ignored in order to create physical science were dramatically included by the great nineteenth-century physiologists, and the reassembling continues to this day. In neuroscience today we are at the frontier of this steady advance of physical science—now we are extending the philosophical revolution of the seventeenth century and exploring the relationship of brain activities to human intention and behavior. To find scientifically successful methods of relating physics to observable biological phenomena, in the next chapter we examine historical examples that have found ways for utilizing physical science without falling into the oversimplifications of deductive science.

NOTES

1. For a clear discussion of Galileo's philosophy, science, and life, see David Wooten (2010). *Galileo: Watcher of the skies.* New Haven: Yale University Press.
2. Galileo Galilei. (2008). Knowing properties vs. knowing essences. In M. A. Finocchiaro (Ed. & Trans.), *The essential Galileo* (p. 101). Indianapolis: Hackett Publishing Company.
3. Whitehead, A. N. (1975). *A philosopher looks at science* (p. 63). New York: Philosophical Library.
4. A comprehensive account of Descartes' life and his scientific and philosophical contributions can be found in Clarke, D. M. (2006). *Descartes: A biography.* Cambridge: Cambridge University Press.

5. Descartes, R. (1996). In D. Weismann (Ed.), *Discourse on method and meditations on first philosophy.* New Haven & London: Yale University Press.

6. Ibid. (p. 21).

7. Ibid. (p. 22).

8. For a discussion of Descartes' contributions to science, see Clarke, D. M. (1992). Descartes' philosophy of science and the Scientific Revolution. In J. Cottingham (Ed.), *The Cambridge companion to Descartes* (p. 258). Cambridge: Cambridge University Press.

9. See Jolley, N. (1992). The reception of Descartes' philosophy. In J. Cottingham (Ed.), *The Cambridge companion to Descartes* (p. 393). Cambridge: Cambridge University Press.

10. For an up-to-date but traditional philosophical description of dualism and materialism see Searle, J. R. (1994). *The rediscovery of mind* (pp. 27–57). Cambridge: A Bradford Book, The MIT Press.

11. Nagel, T. (1986). *The view from nowhere* (p. 1). New York: Oxford University Press.

12. Ibid. (p. 3).

13. For a review of Descartes' influence on the invention of the mind, see Rorty, R. (1979). *Philosophy and the mirror of nature* (pp. 17–69). Princeton: Princeton University Press. These pages articulate the traditional philosophical invention of the mind, following Descartes, and establish the criteria for the pragmatist's position that these contingent concepts should be used only when they are useful for understanding and dealing with the world. One central theme of the present volume is that the concepts of mind are not turning out to be valuable in formulating and interpreting neuroscientific experiments, particularly in neuroimaging, and therefore it is desirable to study brain function without resorting to those descriptions.

14. Janik, A., & Toulmin, S. (1973). *Wittgenstein's Vienna* (pp. 211–227). Chicago: Ivan R. Dee, discusses the complexities of Wittgenstein's relation with the Vienna Circle of positivists. In their reading, the Tracticus was misinterpreted by the Vienna Circle as supporting its goals of finding logical explanations of the world, while Wittgenstein's sense of its achievements was that it had shown that such explanations were limited to logic and mathematics. "When the logical positivism of the Vienna Circle was taking shape, the philosophers and scientists involved deeply respected the authority of Wittgenstein and his Tracticus. Yet he remained an on-looker and an increasingly skeptical one...[because]...they were turning an argument designed to circumvent all philosophical doctrines into a source of new doctrines, meanwhile leaving the original difficulties unresolved" (p. 215). In 1927 Wittgenstein agreed to meet with Carnap and other members of the Vienna Circle, "but it immediately became apparent that their positions were far apart—perhaps unbridgeably so." Janik and Toulmin quote Wittgenstein's good friend Paul Engellmann: "A whole generation of disciples was able to take Wittgenstein as a positivist, because he has something of enormous importance in common with the positivists: he draws the line between what we can speak about and what we must be silent about just as they do. The difference is only that they have nothing to be silent about."

15. Ibid. (p. 198)

16. Rorty, R. (1989). *Contingency, irony, and solidarity* (p. 4). Cambridge: Cambridge University Press.
17. Ibid. (p. 5)
18. Rorty, R. (1999). Davidson's mental–physical distinction. In L. E. Hahn (1999). The philosophy of Donald Davidson (p. 576). *The Library of Living Philosophers,* vol. XXVII. Chicago and LaSalle, IL: Southern Illinois University at Carbondale.
19. Ibid. (p. 583).
20. Wittgenstein, L. (1960). *The Blue and Brown Books* (p. 7). New York: Harper & Row.
21. Bennett, M. R., & Hacker, P. M. S. (2003). *Philosophical foundations of neuroscience* (p. 29). Malden, MA: Blackwell Publishers.
22. Ibid. (p. 29).
23. Ibid. (p. 243).

4

Neuroscience

A Multidisciplinary, Multilevel Field

Neuroscience is a multilevel, multidisciplinary subject comprising morphological, functional, and physical studies of the central nervous system. The challenge for neuroscience has been to relate the objective explanations of brain activity offered by physical science to observable behavior without relying on theories that are reductive of the brain's complexity—and deductive in their acceptance of "everyday" assumptions about mental processes. Phenomena in neuroscience, as diverse as action potentials and the person in the state of consciousness, can be identified by mechanisms and properties at different levels—at the neuronal and cellular level for the former and at the behavioral level for the latter. In the following chapters, I distinguish between the observable fact that a person is in the state of consciousness from an interest in defining the mental activities that are purported to underlie that observation. Once phenomena are identified as observable processes, they are open to exploration by different disciplines, ranging from the microscopic concern with potentials, ions, and energetics to the complex human level, where reliable data are obtained from behavior and the person's responses. I will argue that different levels of scientific investigation require different methods, techniques, and assumptions, and that there are no normative ways to conduct interdisciplinary, multilevel studies. In other words, I will propose that if one is studying frogs, one would use one set of tools to track the fluid mechanics of how the frog swims in the water, another to track the mating rituals, another to track mutations in frog species over time, another to understand the frog's digestive system, and so on.

Multidisciplinary, multilevel investigations of interdisciplinary research have recently been formulated as a general epistemology—called the philosophy of mechanisms—that is useful in studying biological phenomena.[1-3] As discussed briefly in the introductory chapter, and in more detail below, this method does not seek general laws that provide a single explanation of a phenomenon but rather favors investigating the many properties and mechanisms that contribute to it. The resulting set of mechanisms or properties necessary for the phenomenon to occur can be considered as forming a mosaic that surrounds the phenomenon with contributing mechanisms. This is the kind of understanding that biologists generally seek rather than a reducing law. In this chapter we review several historical examples of bridging studies that have identified mechanisms and made correlations across levels and between disciplines that are relevant for the interdisciplinary problems posed in neuroscience. As a background to my proposal that neuroscience seeks a complex and multilevel appreciation of the varieties of brain activity rather than seeking to reduce brain chemistry and human activity to one unified theory, we turn to analogous historical examples of interdisciplinary explanations from evolutionary biology and quantum physics.

THE UNITY OR DISUNITY OF SCIENCE

Before inquiring what contributions the many disciplines of neuroscience can make to questions about the brain and its role in behavior, we must first ask what kind of answer can be expected. Are there universal laws of physics that hold across levels, or does each level require its own kind of explanation? To pose such questions is to enter an ongoing philosophical controversy about the scope and unity of scientific knowledge. Cognitive Neuroscience is one of the disciplines based on the assumption that science is of a unity and proposes that universally understood logical activities of a computer-like brain can provide the means of defining our individual psyches. On the other hand, advocates of the disunity of science, of whom there are many, respond that different levels of organized matter—elementary particles, atoms, molecules, solids, and so on, all the way up to the complexities of people and societies—present phenomena that require different means of understanding.

Proposals to explain observations at all levels, from the nuclear to the human, by overarching general laws have been made by physicists, emboldened by the successes of their laws in explaining the inorganic world. In explaining their theories eminent physicists have emphasized methodological differences coming from the perspectives of their different subfields of physics. In his book *Dreams of a Final Theory*, Steven Weinberg, a theorist of great renown in elementary particle physics, posits the existence of a universal theory "that would be of unlimited validity and entirely satisfying in its completeness and consistency."[4] Such a theory, he claims, would explain how all scientific knowledge is connected. On the other hand, the distinguished condensed-matter theorist Phillip Anderson has shown that although the quantum laws for elementary particles have high symmetry, their symmetry is "broken," even at the level of small molecules, by chemical forces that hold a molecule in one particular isomeric form rather than in an equivalent symmetrical state allowed by quantum laws.[5] Since elementary laws are not sufficient to explain molecular properties even at this simple level, Anderson argues that more complex and less symmetrical levels of social science or psychology can never be explained by laws of elementary particles. However, Anderson goes on to claim that laws can be found; they will be new generalizations based on specific sets of experimental and theoretical discoveries characteristic of the different levels of organized matter. Despite their disagreement about methods of relating to data, Weinberg and Anderson have much in common. Both assert that laws can be found at all levels, from molecules to individual humans to the social sciences, although they differ about the variables in the laws. The differences in their proposed laws derive from their procedures for finding them. Weinberg believes, in principle and with practical reservations, in an all-encompassing final theory derived from particle physics, while Anderson would reformulate each field's data empirically to generate general theories that would be consistent with the laws of physics. Both men have demonstrated in their careers the power of theoretical concepts in physics. However, in more heuristic fields such as economics and the other sciences of human behavior, they both seek the kind of general law whose value I am questioning. In contrast to these appeals for a unified view of science in which reducing laws are seen as having determinate power at all levels and for all disciplines, I turn to several histories of science, where interdisciplinary understanding has been found in lieu of such unifying theories.

In a collection of essays, 16 authors have presented compelling criticisms of the unity of science.[6] Most reject reductionism as a unifying principle, on the grounds that to reduce one subject to another represents an outmoded and failed positivistic attempt at unification. Many of the authors are attracted instead by the "village" concept of science, according to which separate communities grow up around a given topic, interacting only occasionally. This patchwork-quilt definition posits a heterogeneous, multidisciplinary, time- and place-dependent description of science. The book's introduction frames the debate:

"Most of the authors here begin with the view that there is something local about scientific knowledge and then try to explore where that intuition leads.... What are the philosophical consequences of a dis-unified science? The disunity (or unity) of science is fiercely contested ground because these attributes of homogeneity and diversity are so deeply tied to the images of authority of the sciences."[7]

Communication between the different disciplines within science—in other words, interdisciplinary studies—is the subject of an essay in this collection by Ian Hacking. He notes that scientists, in an attempt "to find connections between important phenomena that have hitherto seemed independent,"[8] have embraced the goal of integration and harmony. In Hacking's view, the search for unifying concepts reflects the beliefs held by scientists like Faraday, who spent 20 years before finding a connection between magnetism and electricity, and Einstein, who never stopped trying to reconcile gravity with quantum mechanics.

Hacking finds that metaphysical descriptions of the world, in the closed forms that philosophers (and theoretical physicists) use, are inadequate. At the same time, he accepts that the world "may be made of facts...but...is not a ragbag of facts,"[9] a description he attributes to Wittgenstein. Nor does he go to the other extreme of asserting that there is a fundamental "structure to the truths about the world." Hacking recognizes that physicists like Faraday believed that "phenomena of roughly the same level of generality are connected to each other,"[10] and that each influences the other. Hence, he concludes, the successes of physics in unifying many apparently distinct findings support a search for connections of "harmonious integration, not singleness."[11] Making connections between phenomena from different disciplines is a way of describing interdisciplinary research that is discussed from several perspectives in this chapter. Connections are not explanations of one field by another, nor are they reductions of one to another; they are correlations of the differing properties of a phenomenon that are recognized by considerations from more than one perspective.

Hacking speaks of different disciplines as employing different styles of scientific reasoning. Each style "has its own self-stabilizing techniques," but some are "more effective than others." This provides a basis for judging interdisciplinary science that is consistent with the spectrum of differing reliability across disciplines, as introduced by Rorty.[12] The subjects for which connections are being made in cognitive neuroscience—psychology, computer science, and physical science—have been developed by different methods of scientific reasoning. Since each has resulted in a body of knowledge with enough empirical validity to be considered science, Hacking, with the detachment of a historian, can claim that all these methods are successful because they are self-authenticating. But the levels of reliability offered by different scientific fields are not the same since they deal with different issues. Quantitative experimental support allows the claims of physics, astronomy, and chemistry to be more dependable—they can build bridges and telephones—than theories of the social sciences because of the intrinsic complexity of humans. The greater reliability of physical theories is a matter of degree. Cognitive Neuroscience earned substantial admiration because it aimed to increase the reliability of a psychological theory by offering testable predictions, thereby promising to harden a softer, more interpretive social science into a field that fell further along Rorty's gamut where more precise consensus could be garnered. But the influences of social context and scientific environment on the search for truth in human sciences (like neuroscience) are becoming more evident because of the pioneering work of Ludwik Fleck.

SCIENCE AS THE PRODUCT OF THOUGHT COLLECTIVES

A description of neuroscience that accepts its heterogeneity can build on Fleck's studies of the genesis of a scientific fact. Born in Lvov, Poland, in 1896, Fleck was a professional immunologist who wrote about his subject from a historical and social perspective.[13] He saw the everyday practice of science as a dynamic, evolving subject dominated by social-psychological "thought styles" (similar to Kuhn's subsequent description of paradigms). These guiding styles have been described by Barbara Herrnstein Smith as "systems of ideas and assumptions and related perceptual, classificatory and behavioral dispositions that prevail among the members of particular epistemic communities."[14] Fleck called these communities "thought collectives." Smith's summary and analysis of Fleck calls attention to this hitherto underappreciated, innovative scientist-philosopher.

In Fleck's epistemology, for a scientific truth or fact to exist there must be a "thought collective" of individuals with shared values and knowledge who can accept it. Without the common opinions, attitudes, and styles of thought that bind these individuals together, a concept would either be unclear or be understood differently. Fleck asserted that "Truth is not a convention but rather, in historical perspective, an event in the history of thought."[15] The dependence of scientific facts on time and place contrasts with the so-called Whig history of science, in which the "discovery" of scientific facts obscures social, individual, and cognitive interactions involved in the emergence of a finding. Fleck tried to uncover the contingent contributions by what he termed "comparative epistemology," which "traced the historical emergence and development of acts in their intellectual and social contexts." He emphasized the continually changing nature of science—how any result is "the starting point for new lines everywhere developing and again joining up with others. Nor do the old lines remain unchanged.... This network in continuous fluctuation is called reality or truth."[16] Smith contrasts this quote with the epigraph of Popper's *Logic of Scientific Discovery*[17] (published the same year as Fleck's *Genesis and Development of a Scientific Fact*): "Theories are nets: only he who casts will catch." She continues, "For Popper, the net, an individually conceived conjecture, may catch truth. For Fleck, the net, a web of shifting, intersecting beliefs and practices, *is* truth."[18]

To Galileo's relation of observer and object, Fleck adds a third factor: the "existing fund of knowledge" in a field. This fund, he says, constitutes "a basic factor of all new knowledge." For Fleck, as later for Rorty and Kuhn, that which is accepted as truth is what works within a thought collective and which changes with the results it helps to create and from the changes in its society. Just as there is no absolute criterion of fitness for evolutionary survival, so too, he wrote, there is no general criterion for what is accepted as truth outside of the intellectual environments in which these truths emerged and the history to which they were adapted.

The heterogeneous nature of neuroscience makes it all the more important to recognize the role played by Fleck's thought collectives and their dependence on the changing ideas accepted at different times. Fleck identified the heterogeneity and historical dependence of understanding by studying the changing epistemology of syphilis. Selecting "one of the best established medical facts: the fact that the so-called Wasserman reaction is related to syphilis," he asked, "How did this empirical fact originate and in what does it consist?"[19] He traced the understanding of this disease from the fifteenth century, when it was lumped with undifferentiated skin symptoms frequently localized in the genitals, to the present germ-based Wasserman theory. He developed the validity of comparative epistemology that I propose can illuminate the historical perceptions of mental life by considering neuroscience as an assembly of thought collectives with a common interest in the brain but whose ability to communicate is limited by their different backgrounds. Focusing on the assumptions and empirical results in different thought collectives, we possibly can, by realizing their historical dimensions, disentangle contributions from different disciplines to neuroscience. For example, it might help, in planning neuroimaging experiments, to realize that ideas of mental activities persisting since Descartes could profit from incorporating modern empiricism. Just as modern chemistry has replaced the alchemist's goals of transforming lead to gold while retaining many of their empirical distinctions; modern brain science need not be committed to healing Descartes' intractable division of mind and matter while dealing with their indirect symptoms.

MOLECULAR GENETICS AND EVOLUTIONARY BIOLOGY

The attempt to establish connections between different levels in biology can be illustrated by examining the relationship between molecular biology and its partner, evolutionary biology. Qualitative differences between the observational methods of Darwin's evolutionary theory and the well-established experimental nature of physical theory have allowed evolutionary biologists to reflect upon their science, since both evolutionary biology and the more physically based science of genetics have studied heritability, an important factor in natural selection.

No scientist has made a greater contribution in this area than Ernst Mayr. In his long and distinguished career, Mayr (simultaneously with other participations in the great synthesis) incorporated modern molecular studies of genetics into evolutionary theory, thereby strengthening Darwin's postulates of heritability. Until this synthesis, heritability, although central, was merely an assumption of evolutionary biology. Mayr showed how a philosophy of biology could reconcile the observable, molecular contributions of genetics with the large-scale theories of evolution. Paradoxically, his first step toward reconciling these disparate methodologies was to deny their unity in biology. Mayr asserted that "systems at each hierarchical level have two properties. They act as wholes (as though they were a homogeneous entity), and their characteristics cannot be deduced (even in theory) from the most complete knowledge of the components."[20] Furthermore, Mayr claimed that not all characteristics of the whole can be predicted from the individual components.

The separation of the whole from its parts can be understood only by reconciling the different methods used to study each. The whole—the organism that has survived evolutionary pressures—is studied by comparison and observation, producing results that are historical, not quantitative, and embodied in what Mayr called theories rather than in predictive laws. On the other hand, components such as genetics are studied by the experimental methods of classical physical science and have quantitative predictions. Mayr contended that the roles of the experimental and comparative methods can be understood only if one realizes that biology draws upon two rather different major fields of study: the biology of proximate causations (broadly, functional or molecular biology) and the biology of ultimate causations (evolutionary biology).

Mayr's first-order division of evolutionary biology prescribes dissimilar methods that reflect their individual strengths for the study of different topics. However, the separation between these two aspects of biology is not the end of the story. Biologists do not follow a strict bottom-up (functional) or top-down (evolutionary) methodology. They are, and should be, opportunistic, choosing freely from either approach to develop an understanding of how things work. In that search, evolutionary concepts, such as the efficiency or the survival value of the mechanism, play different roles than, for example, the quantitative laws of

Mendelian genetics. Although the gap between ultimate and proximate causations is hardly as wide as that between subjective states of human consciousness and the objectivity of physical science, the ultimate causes proffered by evolutionary theory are still significantly less amenable to quantitative testing than the laws of a proximate science such as genetics. The modern great synthesis of Darwinian evolutionary theory and modern genetics illustrates the understanding that can be achieved by connecting components of the two fields. As Mayr has shown, suitable methods must first provide reliable understandings of the separate parts. Then, and only then, can the parts be combined to describe sections of the whole.

A recent article on the ecology and evolution of antibiotic-resistant bacteria explores the many benefits that accrue from combining the fields of evolutionary concepts and molecular genetics. Bergstrom and Feldgarden[21] studied the development of bacterial antibiotic resistance, starting with the widespread increase in hospital-acquired bacterial infections. More than 200,000 cases are reported every year in the United States alone, resulting in at least 90,000 mortalities. (Estimates range as much as ten times higher.) The appearance of antibiotic resistance coincided with the discovery of antibiotics: bacteria resistant to penicillin, the first antibiotic, appeared within 1 year after its first clinical use in 1943.

Bergstrom and Feldgarden surveyed the genetic mechanisms for the development of resistance to ten of the most commonly used antibiotics and identified three distinct genetic accommodations: point mutations, homologous recombination of existing point mutants, and heterologous recombination of novel resistant loci. The variety of survival mechanisms they discovered was astonishing, and the value of their understanding for controlling the spread of drug resistance demonstrated the power of bringing physical science of molecular genetics to bear on evolutionary populations. In bringing evolutionary biology and genetics to bear on their question they show the benefits accruing to the thought collective that Mayr created in which these two disciplines were harnessed to move understanding forward.

Evolutionary biology and molecular genetics are two disciplines studying living processes with different origins that have been developed during their histories. Their methods, dependent on the level of their subject matter, necessarily have different degrees of objectivity and reliability. The relative importance of subjective and objective factors is apparent from the level of their subject. An analogous interplay of subjective and objective elements in physics was long unrecognized, only becoming evident by the quantum revolution, when the claims of classical physics for objectivity were curtailed by the uncertainty principle.

MULTILEVELS IN QUANTUM PHYSICS

In the early years of the twentieth century, the revolutionary scientific discoveries of quantum mechanics brought the issue of subjectivity versus objectivity to the fore. The novel findings of quantum physics demanded that certainty, the objective basis of classical physics, must be abandoned at the quantum level. The Heisenberg uncertainty principle showed that there are inescapable minima for the combined uncertainties of conjugate coordinates such as energy and time or position and momentum. Therefore we cannot know the simultaneous position and momentum of a particle; it is impossible to calculate exactly where it will be and what it will be doing in the future. The Schrodinger wave equation responded to this uncertainty at the quantum level by allowing the *probable* values of these parameters to be statistically described. In this way, physical phenomena at the quantum level continue to be investigated with great usefulness by quantum mechanics without dependence on the causal relations of classical physics.

Classical mechanics was based on a separation between the observer and the object under study. The expectations in classical physics were that separate observations of a phenomenon like an electron, by different observers using different methods (responding, for example, to waves rather than particles), could be integrated into an explanation of its nature. By integrating the observations from different perspectives this explanation would introduce an objective understanding of the phenomenon. However, quantum uncertainty did not allow the results of wave and particle experiments to be integrated so as to describe the electron as a particle at a measured position traveling with a measured velocity that would be objective, independent of the observer. In the world of quantum physics, the results of an experiment were limited to describing the electron as either a wave or a particle, depending on the observer's subjective choice of experimental method.

Bohr's theory of complementarity asserted that a description of the experimental measurements and their results exhausts our knowledge of the phenomenon. Complementarity states that measurements made by human-scale instruments describe all that we can know about the electron and other quantum phenomena.[22] Quantum uncertainty undermined the possibility of finding an objective understanding of subatomic phenomenon (i.e., of combining the wave and particle properties of an electron so as to predict the future values of its position and momentum). In the microscopic world, Heisenberg's uncertainty prevailed, but Bohr accepted that we knew this world through measurements that presented information in terms of classical physics. By measuring the wavelike nature of the electron, we could characterize its wave properties of frequency and velocity. On the other hand, measuring the electron's particle-like nature in photoelectric emission would enable us to describe it as a particle with a specified mass and momentum. Both wave and particle measurements could be made with human-size equipment and the values of the particle or wave could be displayed on laboratory-sized readouts, but the views from the different subjective measurements could not be combined to describe a particle with objective properties.

Bohr struggled with the inadequacy of everyday language to describe the understanding offered by quantum physics. Far from restricting our efforts to put questions to nature in the form of experiments, he asserted that the notion of complementarity merely characterized the answers that such enquiries can be expected to yield. Bohr claimed that by accepting what we can know from physical experimentation and thereby sacrificing the older standards of cause and effect, we reach the best available objective understanding of physical results. In his words:

> From our present standpoint, physics is to be regarded not so much as the study of something a priori given, but rather as the development of methods for ordering and surveying human experience. In this respect our task must be to account for such experience in a manner independent of individual subjective judgment and objective in the sense that it can be unambiguously communicated in the common human language.[23]

Bohr's thoughts were complex, as quantum physics required. Extrapolated to biology, I believe that they provide a useful guide for neuroscience—a guide that, like complementarity itself, is apparently contradictory. Bohr pointed to a biological complementarity that finds the fullest available understanding of the relations between neuronal activity and behavior in simultaneously accepting experimental observations of behavioral and neurophysiological phenomena without trying to unify them. He saw that complementarity has given us a new background for discussing "notions beyond the language of physics."[24] In speaking of the value of complementarity for biology, he emphasized that complementarity helps us to understand "the way in which our whole conceptual framework has developed from serving the more primitive necessities of daily life to coping with knowledge gained by systematic scientific research. Thus, as long as the word 'life' is retained for practical or epistemological reasons the dual approach in biology will surely persist."[24] Just as the phenomena of an "electron" cannot be described by unifying its properties, so too have terms describing life at the organismic level, including mental processes presumed to underlie behavior, like mind, memory, and attention, lost the possibility of being described by integrating observations at the behavioral and neuronal level. Long-established concepts of mental processes that have been so useful in their respective domains that they have seemed to be innately understood cannot, according to biological complementarity, be meaningfully discussed in neuroscience. The basis for a community's understanding of the terms happen at different levels; they occur as "truths" to different communities.

Just as Bohr attempted to come to terms with the loss of causal explanations, a precious expectation in classical physics, so experimentation has forced us to propose limits to the utility of the Cartesian concept of an immaterial "mind" that is available to introspection. It is a sobering limitation of science to accept that the idea that this "mind"—a familiar and useful concept that pervades our daily lives—will not be explained by physical brain science (e.g., neuroimaging) in the foreseeable future, if ever. This position, comparing the loss of our everyday certainty about mind with loss of the long-established causality in classical physics, leads us to apply Bohr's solution to neuroscience. Following William James's warning that naming something does not mean that we have found it to be real in any useful way, neuroscience should not seek to find brain activities that explain the cognitive concepts that psychology in Western culture assumed were part of nature. Nor is there reason to believe that differently formulated assumptions about the nature of mental processes, such as networks, or a more accurate use of language or a theory of brain connectivity will be any better fused with brain activities. Complementarity, introduced to reconcile the loss of causality at the quantum level, proposes that the totality of our understanding is based on the observations made from different perspectives. By the same token, although physical studies of brain activities do not explain the hypothetical concepts of cognitive psychology postulated to underlie an observable behavior, such as consciousness, they can be correlated with measurable aspects of that behavior indicating that the person is, for example, in the state of consciousness. There is value to be gained by examining a topic from these different viewpoints with different tools—as the work of Fleck, Mayr, and Bohr has served to illustrate. However, showing that an observable, physical, neuronal activity is a necessary property of the person who is displaying an observable, measurable behavior is fundamentally different from saying that neuroscience is capable of defining mental abstractions like consciousness in terms of neurons and molecules. As Bohr observed, "It is wrong to think that the task of physics is to find out how nature is. Physics concerns what we can say about nature."[25] Analogously, the task of neuroscience is not to answer questions about brain function posed by philosophers or cognitive psychologists, but rather to measure what we can and cannot say about brain activity. Neuroscience can help us define the questions we can ask with the hope of finding a meaningful answer. Science is able to define some necessary properties that both the electron and the person's brain must possess in order to fit the observables. An electron must be capable of being diffracted by a grating, while a functioning midtemporal cortex is necessary for a person to remember incidents from a distant past; however, we do not have, in either case, the necessary and *sufficient* conditions that would provide the kind of objective explanation that we are proposing is unattainable in both cases.

THE MOSAIC OF MECHANISMS

I have been emphasizing how Pragmatism allows us to judge the relevance of hypotheses about mental life by their usefulness for experiments. For Pragmatists the value of a hypothesis is to be determined by the results it can generate. In being guided by scientific usefulness, Pragmatism has much in common with a recent direction in philosophy of science, particularly of neuroscience, that has aimed "to construct a model of explanation that reflects, rather than merely accommodates, the structure of explanations in neuroscience."[26] This naturalized philosophy of biology that takes its standards from what scientists actually do to understand biological function has been called, because of the methodology it proposes, a philosophy of Mechanisms. This philosophy starts not by prescribing what neuroscientists should do but by examining what they in fact do, when looking for explanations. As Carl Craver states, "in neuroscience, as opposed to physics or chemistry, three main features of explanation demand attention: (1) explanations describe mechanisms; (2) explanations span multiple levels" and (3) explanations would integrate findings from multiple fields by simply listing them.[27] This field systematizes the several conclusions I have reached from historical examples and in the choice of Pragmatism over alternative philosophies. We are not to seek explanation of a phenomenon, such as the action potential, at a single level. Rather, we begin to understand what it is when we see its activities described by mechanisms at different levels in neuroscience: intracellular electrical measurements, vesicular exocytosis, ion maintenance of membrane potential, neurotransmitter fluxes and recycling, energy consumption or work done as ATP hydrolysis—all contribute to a composite understanding of the action potential that grows as it is extended to more levels and disciplines. Craver calls this understanding achieved by multidisciplinary study a *mosaic*.[28] In this composite view of a phenomenon, the constraints on a mechanism obtained at different levels and by different disciplines provide as comprehensive a view as possible for understanding the characteristically multilevel phenomena of interest to neuroscience. In the mosaic model an understanding is obtained not by reduction of a phenomenon from a higher level to a more fundamental level but rather by "using results from different fields to constrain a multilevel mechanistic explanation."[29] Craver is particularly resistant to the traditional descriptions in Cognitive Neuroscience in which the highest levels of conceptualization, such as memory, are reduced to a mechanism at a more fundamental level such as neurons or molecules. Mechanistic philosophy claims that neuroscientists do not completely accept either the bottom-up approach, which proposes to explain biological functions from the interactions and properties of its component parts, or the top-down view, which starts with a systemic description. Mechanisms come from many levels and there is no single fundamental level of explanation. The cumulative picture of a phenomenon in which complementarity between conclusions achieves a rough sort of unity, obtained as the mosaics multiply, is responsible for the robust understandings of neuroscience. In an example of mechanistic studies satisfying this philosophy, Craver describes the many levels on which long-term potentiation (LTP) has been studied.[30] This phenomenon, in which synapses that have once fired in response to a stimulus are more easily fired thereafter, has been studied by mechanisms at different levels. The relationship of LTP to the organism's act of remembering is realized in the behavior of mice struggling to remember a maze, while on the brain level the mechanisms of LTP include the activities of the hippocampus during a rat's movement through a maze, and on the cellular and molecular levels LTP involves synaptic and molecular activity during that behavior. Invoking mechanisms at different levels and disciplines is in accord with Hacking's emphasis on making connections to explain phenomena, and Bohr's notion of the limitations on understanding defined by complementarity.

UNDERSTANDING AT THE LEVEL OF METABOLISM

The Pragmatic philosophy that I advocate for neuroscience has much in common with the mosaic of understanding to be found by mechanisms from different disciplines at different levels. The example in the following pages shows how brain activities support the person in a state of consciousness. We connect certain brain activities that are at work when a person is known to be in that state because of his behavior with activities at the neuronal level, but we do not use neuronal activities to explain the behavior. More emphatically, we do not use them to explain some mental concept that has been proposed to be the basis of the behavior.

Craver is careful to explain that the mosaics obtained from mechanisms or properties provide only a methodological skeleton for understanding in neuroscience. The levels at which mechanisms are found and the actual nature of the mechanisms that are to be fitted into this skeleton will vary with the needs of the problem and with the availability of scientific resources.

He quite understandably leaves it to the neuroscientist to decide which levels and which methods are valuable for any phenomenon.

Insights offered by different mechanisms depend not only on their relevance to the phenomenon but also upon the reliability and scope of the disciplines where the mechanisms are developed. The strictures of relevance and reliability support a high value for the usefulness of brain metabolism in neuroscience. *In vivo* MRS, calibrated blood oxygen level dependent (BOLD), and electrophysiological experiments provide valuable jumping-off points for correlating physical and higher-level systemic processes. Results from these new experimental methods have been relating information available from bench-top chemistry and physiology, and the measured rates of purified enzymes, to rates of metabolic pathways measured *in vivo*.

The following chapter will uncover mechanisms of brain energy consumption and relate them to neuronal activity by *in vivo* metabolic experiments. These mechanisms of brain work will subsequently be correlated with observable human behavior.

NOTES

1. Bechtel, W. (2009). *Mental mechanisms: Philosophical perspectives on cognitive neuroscience.* New York: Psychology Press, Taylor & Francis Group.
2. Machamer, P., Darden, L., & Craver, C. F. (2000). Thinking about mechanisms. *Philosophy of Science, 67,* 1–25.
3. Craver, C. F. (2007). *Explaining the brain: Mechanisms and the mosaic unity of neuroscience.* New York: Oxford University Press.
4. Weinberg, S. (1994). *Dreams of a final theory, the scientist's search for the ultimate laws of nature.* New York: Vintage Books, Random House.
5. Anderson, P. W. (1972). More is different. *Science, 69,* 1097–1099.
6. Galison, P., & Stump, D. J. (Eds., 1996). *The disunity of science: Boundaries, contexts, and power.* Stanford: Stanford University Press.
7. Ibid. (p. 2).
8. Hacking, I. (1996). In P. Galison & D. J. Stump (Eds.), *The disunity of science: Boundaries, contexts, and power* (p. 43). Stanford: Stanford University Press.
9. Ibid. (p. 49).
10. Ibid. (p. 49).
11. Ibid. (p. 57).
12. Rorty, R. (1999). Davidson's mental–physical distinction. In L. E. Hahn (1999). *The philosophy of Donald Davidson* (p. 576). The Library of Living Philosophers, vol. XXVII. Chicago and LaSalle, IL: Southern Illinois University at Carbondale.
13. Fleck, L. (1979). *Genesis and development of a scientific fact.* Chicago: The University of Chicago Press.
14. Smith, B. H. (2005). *Scandalous knowledge: Science, truth and the human* (p. 49). Durham, NC: Duke University Press.

15. Op. cit., Fleck (p. 100).

16. Ibid. (p. 79).

17. Popper, K. [1935] (1965) *The logic of scientific discovery.* Rev. ed., no trans. given. New York: Harper and Row.

18. Op. cit., Smith (p. 51).

19. Op. cit., Fleck (p. xxviii).

20. Mayer, E. (1988). *A new philosophy of biology* (p. 15). Cambridge: Harvard University Press.

21. Bergstrom, C. T., & Feldgarden, M. (2008). The ecology and evolution of antibiotic-resistant bacteria. In S. C. Sterns & J. C. Koella (Eds.), *Evolution in health and disease* (2nd ed., pp. 125–137). New York: Oxford University Press.

22. Pais, A. (1991). *Niels Bohr's times in physics, philosophy, and polity* (pp. 224–232). Oxford: Clarendon Press.

23. Bohr, N. (1987). *The philosophical writings of Niels Bohr, Vol. III: Essays 1958–1962 on atomic physics and human knowledge* (p. 10). Woodbridge, CT: Ox Bow Press.

24. Ibid. (p. 21).

25. Petersen, A. (1963). Philosophy of Niels Bohr. *Bulletin of Atomic Scientists,* xix:8–14.

26. Op. cit., Craver (p. x).

27. Ibid. (p. 27).

28. Ibid. (pp. 228–271).

29. Ibid. (p. 231).

30. Ibid. (pp. 236–244).

5

The State of Cognitive Neuroscience

An Over-Optimistic Theory

With the growth of neuroimaging methods like fMRI and PET, enthusiastic researchers (both from within and outside of neuroscience) proposed theories about brain function that asserted these physical methods could identify brain activities at a rational level and could thus provide rigorous causal explanations for everyday phenomena. However, while neuroimaging experiments did indeed open new areas of brain studies, creating an empirical field with informative results and still-greater promise, it soon became apparent that they failed to find these causal explanations of everyday phenomena. Despite an ongoing absence of experimental support, the appeal of these theoretical expectations has been so great that imaging results continue to be interpreted in terms of its goals. Consequently, superb modern methods and valuable experimental findings are intermingled with unreliable interpretations and claims that form a muddle as to what can be expected from neuroimaging. This chapter focuses on the original claims of the most promising of these theories—Cognitive Neuroscience—and shows how specific experimental programs have fallen far short of supporting expectations, and how reformulations and reinterpretations of the data have created confusion as to whether or not the original goals are being met. By identifying and removing the original claims of a rational brain basis for mental concepts, we can distinguish and appreciate the extraordinary achievements and promise of brain imaging as an empirical physical science. To develop the insights into human behavior that can be drawn from noninvasive brain experiments, I will examine some typical results in living humans and in animal models. Since the noninvasive methods of fMRI and MRS measure cerebral energy production and metabolism, we start by describing the role they have played in the recent history of neurophysiology.

Metabolic pathways, particularly those of energy production and consumption that serve the body's physiological needs, have long been the basis for understanding systemic functions. Before the recent biochemical focus on DNA, RNA, and the structures of purified proteins, bodily functions were considered the exclusive province of physiological chemistry. Early neurophysiological research focused on the supply of nutrients to the brain and the electrical activity of neurons. The ability to measure cerebral blood flow (CBF) and metabolism noninvasively has allowed methods such as PET, MRS, and fMRI to become the working tools of brain science. This chapter will trace the development of neurophysiological methods for measuring CBF, energy consumption, and metabolism, starting with early studies on animals and humans. Then uses of neuroimaging techniques proposing to relate mental activities and brain physiology are examined and analyzed. First, however, the physical processes responsible for producing the imaging signals are discussed.

BRAIN ENERGY AND WORK

At a fundamental physical level, the brain interacts with the rest of the body by means of CBF and the transport of metabolites such as glucose and oxygen via the vasculature. Although the human brain constitutes only about 2% of the body's mass, it accounts for approximately 20% of the body's total oxygen consumption. Moreover, it is well established that glucose is the main, indeed almost the only, source of carbon for the brain. It follows that glucose oxidation is the dominant pathway of cerebral energy production.

The delivery of fuels to the brain and their relation to cerebral function form a fascinating research narrative. It starts with the work of Roy and Sherrington,[1] who suggested that there is "an automatic mechanism by which the blood supply of any part of the cerebral tissue is varied in accordance with the activity of the chemical changes which underlie the functional activation of that part." This hypothesis framed the neurophysiological assumption that blood flow, energetics, and neuronal functions are tightly linked. Support for this understanding solidified in the twentieth century, as individual links in the cerebral metabolic chain were studied separately.

Beginning in the 1950s, metabolic rates of glucose and oxygen consumption were evaluated in the whole brain by measuring differences in the arterial (input) and venous (output) concentrations of the metabolites in conjunction with measurements of CBF.[2] These results confirmed and quantified earlier reports establishing the high levels of glucose and oxygen consumption by the brain. The insights resulting from these experiments highlighted the importance of localizing the changes induced in these parameters by stimulation. Earlier measurements by less quantitative methods had reported localized changes, particularly of blood flow, leading researchers to conclude that to some extent localized brain activities could be induced or altered by specific sensory stimuli.[3]

In 1979 Louis Sokoloff, of the National Institutes of Health, pioneered the use of autoradiography to localize activations in animal subjects.[4] He developed methods for infusing radiolabeled analogues of glucose into the brain in such a way that they would be trapped *in situ* instead of being metabolized and carried away by blood flow. The concentrations of these compounds served as a measure of cerebral metabolism—either of the cerebral metabolic rates of glucose (CMR_{glc}) or, with alternative labeled compounds, of CBF. By slicing the extracted brains of sacrificed animals, Sokoloff was able to measure and compare the rates of radioactivity under baseline (nonstimulated) conditions with the changes introduced by stimulation. Sokoloff's methods represented a major step toward modern neuroimaging—they quantified Roy and Sherrington's concept of regional neurovascular coupling. In addition to producing quantitative metabolic information, his autoradiographic experiments revealed an exciting array of **localized** metabolic and blood-flow responses to **sensory** stimulation. Since the experiments examined postmortem brain slices, the method was limited to animals, both awake and anesthetized.

In animal studies of stimulus-induced brain activation, including visual stimulation, limb stimulation, and whisker stimulation,[5] equal fractional changes in CBF and CMR_{glc} were observed. Although localized changes in the cerebral metabolic rate of oxygen (CMR_{O2}) were not measured in these animal studies, the coupled localized increases in CBF and CMR_{glc} during stimulation, considered together with globally averaged values of CMR_{glc} and CMR_{O2}, supported the conclusion that energy was produced by the oxidation of glucose under both nonstimulated *and* stimulated conditions. These studies demonstrated that localized increases in brain energy production, measured from the consumption of glucose (and, implicitly, it was believed, coupled to changes in oxygen consumption), are linked to changes in values of regional CBF.

METHODS FOR LOCALIZING BRAIN ACTIVITY

The extent to which brain activities are localized or delocalized, which has long been a central issue in brain research, is being evaluated by the neuroimaging methods that measure regional changes in neuronal metabolism. To apply autoradiographic methods to humans, noninvasive PET measurements analogous to autoradiography were developed.[6,7] In PET experiments, radiation from radiolabeled metabolites, similar to those used in autoradiography, is measured by a ring of detectors surrounding the head and then mapped to localize specific molecular concentrations. Just as in autoradiography, but actually during the *in vivo* processes, the concentrations of specific labeled compounds allowed metabolic rates to be derived. ^{18}F-fluoro-deoxyglucose was developed as a radioactive tracer to measure changes in CMR_{glc} noninvasively, while CBF was evaluated by measuring the concentration of ^{15}O-water that had flowed into the region. Additional tracers were developed to measure cerebral blood volume (CBV), as well as the oxygen extracted from blood by the brain tissue. The combination of oxygen-extraction, blood-flow, and volume methods enabled changes in CMR_{O2} to be determined by PET and completed its ability to monitor the primary neurophysiological rates.

Soon after these quantitative PET studies of the human brain, fMRI methods were developed and rapidly came to play an important role in functional brain studies.[8-11] In NMR experiments nuclear spins are moved out of their equilibrium state in the magnetic field by radiofrequency waves. The rate at which they return to equilibrium is characterized by a relaxation time, which can be measured and mapped. The fMRI method measures the effects of paramagnetic deoxyhemoglobin on the NMR relaxation times of nearby water protons in the tissue. Since changes in the oxygen level in the blood determine the fraction of hemoglobin in the deoxygenated state, this fMRI imaging method is sometimes called BOLD (blood oxygenation level dependent). The blood oxygen level is the resultant of blood flow, which brings in well-oxygenated arterial blood, and the metabolic activity in the region, which consumes oxygen, creating magnetic deoxygenated hemoglobin. The BOLD results have been analyzed by means of a model that expresses changes in the BOLD signal in terms of the separate incremental changes in CBF and in neuronal energy consumption as measured by CMR_{O2}. The importance for the study of metabolism is that localized values of incremental CMR_{O2} can be derived from measured BOLD signals in the living human when supplemented by measured changes in CBF.

This physiological information will be discussed further in the next chapter. The BOLD fMRI method has high spatial and temporal resolution and is readily measured by slight adaptation of high-field MRI scanners, which are widely available in clinical settings. After the initial demonstration of the fMRI BOLD method in the human brain, the neuroscience community immediately embraced it. The noninvasive nature of fMRI and the fact that it does not require radioactive tracers (which are necessary for PET experiments, thereby limiting the number of experiments allowed) have made it the method of choice in neurobiological studies.[12]

NONINVASIVE LOCALIZATION OF SENSORY STIMULI

In a typical early attempt to localize a functional cerebral response, autoradiography showed that stimulation of a rat's whiskers activated glucose consumption in discrete regions of the brain.[5] I was thrilled by seeing the first autoradiographic results in the early 1980s during a visit to Lou Sokoloff's laboratory. Neurophysiological investigations of neuronal firing, carried out by invasive electrical probing, had shown that cerebral representations of the whiskers, consisting of distinct cylindrical columns of cellular aggregates, are found in a particular region of the brain's somatosensory cortex. These columns, 300 to 500 micrometers in diameter, are called "barrels" because of their shape. Rat's whiskers are sensitive tactile organs: each whisker on the rat snout activates a selected barrel, a correlation that made this system an ideal model for the study of localized functional activity of the central nervous system during stimulation.

A typical fMRI experiment is illustrated by presenting how it produces a map of neuronal activity in the whisker barrel. The fMRI study of rat whisker stimulation was done on living rats, anesthetized to prevent them from moving in the magnet during data acquisition. The fMRI radiofrequency coil, serving as an antenna, surrounds the rat's head, and provision is made for moving one of the animal's several dozen whiskers at a time. Following the BOLD imaging protocol, an image is taken of the head in the absence of stimulation, followed by one taken while a whisker is being tweaked. The first, or baseline, image is then subtracted from the second, or stimulated, image, and the difference signal is evaluated for its statistical significance. Locations of the signals from the cortical barrels have been shown to agree with electrical probes of the brain under similar stimulations.[13] These canonical results, in the deeply anesthetized state required for this experiment, show clearly localized activations of the coupled barrel.

Figure 5.1 illustrates the results of a multislice fMRI experiment,[13] showing the response of the rat brain resulting from touching a single whisker, identified as the D1 whisker on the snout. Whiskers are identified by their position on a rectangular grid, the coordinates being expressed by capital letters and numbers. During stimulation of D1, contralateral activation was observed at a specific position in the sensory cortex. The fMRI location of the D1 whisker barrel agreed perfectly (to within 0.1 mm) with previous locations of this whisker barrel by electrophysiological probing of neuronal firing. The maximum activation was ~0.7 mm below the cortical surface, which was the same depth as the IV cortical layer, known to be the layer of maximum activity. These activations were reproducible both in the same rat and in different animals. A simultaneous stimulation of the D1 and D4 whiskers, monitored by two adjacent coronal imaging slices, showed their separate positions, and the images alternated as each of the whiskers was touched in turn.

The whisker barrel results are typical of the reproducible, noninvasive maps of sensory-induced stimulation that illustrate the powers of fMRI. Numerous detailed, reproducible experiments of the activations produced by visual, auditory, and sensory stimuli have provided similar maps of neurophysiological responses in the brains of living rodents, primates, and humans. These noninvasive maps of responses of the primary sensory pathways to sensory stimuli have generally agreed with earlier invasive results and have extended the scope of

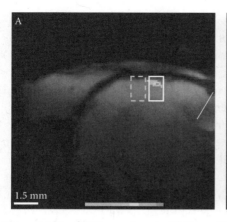
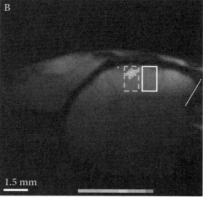

Figure 5.1 An fMRI experiment with D1 and D4 whisker stimulation showing highly localized activation in two contiguous slices. The rat head is slightly tilted to the right, as shown by the orientation of the midline (*white line*). Bar = 1.5 mm. (**A**) Highly located activation was observed ≈4.6 mm from the midline in a coronal plane located ≈2.5 mm posterior to the bregma, corresponding to the anatomical location of D1 barrel. (**B**) Highly localized activation was observed ≈5.4 mm from the midline in a coronal plane located ≈1.5 mm posterior to the bregma, corresponding to the anatomical location of D4 whisker barrel. The dashed yellow rectangle in **A** is the projection of the solid yellow rectangle in **B**, and the dashed white rectangle in *B* is the projection of the solid white rectangle in **A**. In both slices, the rectangles are well separated, suggesting that the observed activation in both slices is individual activation from separate barrels. *Note*: see color insert.

(Reproduced with permission from PNAS. Yang, X., Hyder, F., & Shulman, R. G. (1996). Activation of single whisker barrel in rat brain localized by functional magnetic resonance imaging. *Proceedings of the National Academy of Sciences USA, 93*, 475–478.)

sensory neurophysiology with the noninvasive powers available from magnetic resonance methods. fMRI maps of brain activity during sensory stimulation have extended to the human brain earlier invasive measurements of animals made by electrode probing and have made it possible to map the components of sensory detection. Functional imaging has decomposed human visual inputs into localized activations of motion, color, and intensity[14] that have been identified with analogous regions in the brains of cats and nonhuman primates.[15] It has supported a hierarchical model for visual processing, that has been extended to other sensory stimuli by fMRI experiments on animals and humans.

NEUROIMAGING AND COGNITIVE NEUROSCIENCE

Encouraged by early successes with localizing clearly identified sensory stimulations, researchers used neuroimaging in efforts to describe the cognitive, emotional, and intentional mental concepts of everyday life as localized brain activities. The reproducible responses to sensory stimuli gave rise to expectations that subjective processes and behaviors will be similarly identified and explained by brain activity. In this chapter we examine some general principles underlying this effort and discuss the experimental brain results in two typical efforts to localize higher-order mental concepts.

The intellectual frame for this interpretation was provided by cognitive psychology, and its application to neuroimaging played a significant role in the field of Cognitive Neuroscience. Cognitive Neuroscience, which dominated the interpretations of neuroimaging experiments, was created in the 1970s by fusing a theory of mind from computer science with a traditional philosophical belief in the existence of mental representations of the world. As described by the words of one of its founders, Jerry Fodor, cognitive psychology followed traditional epistemology in assuming that people directly represented to themselves mental processes involved in thinking, learning, and perceiving. The original idea was that cognitive processes are computational—that is, that mental processes can be described as the operation of a computer-like brain on mental representations described by such cognitive concepts as attention, working memory, and word recognition.[16] These distinct components, proposed to be non-overlapping, were called modules. In the Cognitive Neuroscientists' formal definition, the brain response was assumed to reflect these modular psychological inputs; this assumption was derived from earlier psychological experiments in which inserting a behavior increased the subject's time to perform a task, allowing the effects of components to be evaluated. The influence of philosophical assumptions on brain experiments was dramatically revealed by neuroscientists' immediate acceptance, once the methods were available, that images of brain energy consumption and blood flow could answer psychological questions posed by Cognitive Neuroscience.

However, by the early 1980s, it had become evident from experimental results that cognitive psychology presented an oversimplified view of mental activity, and its basic assumptions came under criticism, often expressed as the need for parallel processing. The field survived but did not flourish. However, the development of neuroimaging methods gave Cognitive Neuroscientists new hopes of extending their understanding of brain activity. The ability to image brain activations would play the key role in locating brain responses and correlating them with the modular components of mental activity. In the late 1980s, PET brain maps began to show localized brain activities in response to sensory inputs. As a result, interest in Cognitive Neuroscience rebounded: one picture was more encouraging than a thousand words.

PRIMITIVE DIFFERENCING EXPERIMENTS

The psychological components assembled in the early imaging experiments are described in *Images of Mind* by M. I. Posner and M. E. Raichle.[17] These experiments were implemented by PET, but the procedures were soon adapted, with minor modifications, to fMRI protocols once these methods were available. Posner and Raichle proposed that the performance of a mental task, such as remembering, was represented by the subject as a psychological concept or module, which in this case would be memory, and that imaging experiments could locate where the brain performs memory. For the brain activity to be computer-like it was necessary that both the mental activity and the brain responses be modular, so that the same region would be reproducibly, and uniquely, activated regardless of the behavior in which the mental module was assumed to be imbedded. In other words, they proposed to overcome the subjectivity of mental operations underlying behavior by postulating brain responses that localized an objective representation of the behavior—that is, memory standing for the act of remembering.

Beginning with an analysis of specific behavior, Posner and Raichle proceeded to describe "how scientists study mental operations in objective terms."[18] The first step in their experiments assumed that brain activation during an individual's response to a task, such as pushing a button in response to a question that required a behavior such as remembering or paying attention, would be supported by activations of the postulated memory or attention locations. This assumption was considered plausible because, according to cognitive psychology, individuals thought of the world in generalized, intrinsic, cognitive terms such as memory or attention, rather than in specific terms of observables such as Joseph remembering Mary's face or their infant paying attention to a noise.

It was further assumed that these representations of mental work were modular—that is, that they were the fundamental components or building blocks of mental activities. In many ways, this assumption was the most creative feature of the cognitive psychologists' approach. If true, it identified a level of generalization for mental faculties that fell between the subjective terminology of popular psychology and the more objective language of physiology.

The properties of cognition at both levels—mental representations and measurable brain localizations—were assumed to be modular, located in specific regions or modules and uniquely assignable. Mental activities were assumed to be identified by the modules of cognitive psychology, while their associated brain responses would be found by imaging experiments. A particular cognitive module was assumed always to activate the same brain region, whether presented to the individual in a verbal, visual, or mechanical context. The hierarchical *sensory* inputs were already known to be separable into distinct responses to color, motion, and so forth. The reliable identifications of the sensory stimuli leading to reproducible brain responses were assumed to be the models for cognitive modules. Neuroimaging results were interpreted in attempts to provide support for this model of brain function.

FMRI AND DIFFERENCING EXPERIMENTS

Brain localizations were to be determined in cognitive neuroscience by interpreting the difference map obtained by comparisons of fMRI signals. The tight link between neurophysiological brain regions and the supposed, possible cognitive modules was formalized in the "general linear model" (GLM) by the tensor relationships in statistical parametric mapping.[19] Statistical parametric mapping is widely used for data analysis of fMRI signals to assign a localized brain response to the cognitive module presumed to be introduced by a task. The analogy with the brain responses to sensory stimuli has guided cognitive analysis of functional imaging, and GLM has been built into data interpretation to fulfill this analogy. The connections claimed between postulated psychological modules and the measurable brain volume elements or voxels, when fitted by statistical parametric mapping interpretations of experimental data, can be supported only by the statistical probability that the observed correlations are not due to chance. Support for the objective brain model of cognitive psychology was claimed when a localized brain response to a particular input is unlikely to be a chance occurrence.

MODULARITY AND CONTEXT

The philosophical problem of how to define mental activities and behavior was a primary concern of Ludwig Wittgenstein, who demonstrated that only mathematical or logical terms can be defined unequivocally.[20] Once we recognize, as he did, that even common objects like chairs cannot be rigorously defined, we realize how revolutionary it would be if terms like "working memory" or "attention" could be defined logically and objectively. Initially,[17] the images generated by PET and fMRI and analyzed by the GLM suggested that cognitive neuroscientists could overcome the limitations of the language of folk psychology, with its traditional ways of speaking about familiar mental activities (e.g., believing, remembering, or attending), by indicating explicit physical regions in the brain that corresponded to generalized representations of such activities (i.e., beliefs, memories, or attention). Establishing the brain location of these traditional concepts became a primary goal of functional imaging, in the hope that once the brain responses were identified, they would establish the objectivity of the concepts.

It soon became clear, in contrast to the reliable, modular brain responses to well-defined sensory stimulations, that during the response to higher-level, subjective tasks, other factors are clearly at work. Cognitive neuroimagers have often claimed to locate unique and specific brain responses to behaviors that they described as modules, sometimes going beyond traditional psychological conceptualizations like "memory" or "attention" by using terms from social science such as "rational choice."[21] However, for cognitive modules to have the value in explaining brain activity that was claimed by the original formulation of Cognitive Neuroscience, they must be independent of context. The brain response to a task embodying an activity described by a module such as memory or rational choice must be identical regardless of whether remembering is being used in verbal, motor, or spatial tasks, or whether the rational choice is made in response to arithmetic, financial, or nutritional alternatives. This principle was called into question when it became apparent, as discussed below, that even after modules such as memory were decomposed into components (i.e., working memory, long-term memory, verbal memory, or spatial memory), the brain activations observed continued to depend on the context in which these postulated components were active.

The point being made in this chapter is that the original claims of a rational, computer-like brain that gives modular (i.e., reproducible, localized, scientific) responses to representations of behavior (e.g., memory) are not supported by experiments. One trouble many readers will have with the importance of this point is that they will claim it is almost universally accepted by sophisticated researchers in the field. However, while there is widespread agreement about the limitations of modularity among neuroimagers, there is considerable ambiguity about the possibility of localizing concepts. I do not find that claims of modularity have been unambiguously abandoned and in the two cases discussed in detail below will show how claims of modularity linger even after they have experimentally been rejected, showing that abandoning claims of modularity have not resolved the question but continue to confuse the interpretation of neuroimaging experiments.

The effects of context observed in neuroimaging are not small perturbations of otherwise perfectly reproducible activity, such as could be expected if a computer-like model was a good first approximation of brain function; on the contrary, the effects are large and highly significant, as shown in examples below. Considerable efforts have been made to retain the GLM so as to retain the crucial elements of cognitive psychology. But careful philosophical analysis by Jerry Fodor has shown that the computer-like, rational model of the brain is not working since brain localization of the mental activity presumed to underlie behavior has been experimentally shown to depend on context.[22] Fodor shows that any attempt to explain the observed dependence upon context requires recourse to empirical judgments, which by their very nature destroy the objective, rational, computer-like brain response claimed by Cognitive Neuroscience. In addition to the empirical failing of neuroimaging results, which show the dependence of the proposed modules upon context, attempts to control context or evaluate its contributions are limited by the very uncertainties of the concepts. For example, Fodor notes that the concept of simplicity has very different meanings depending on what is being simplified. Some texts require more explanation in the process of simplification, others less, so that the activities governed by "simplicity" can take opposite forms in different contexts.[23] By the same token, the meaning of "memory" and other such concepts varies according to context in principle as well as experimentally.

Two books by Fodor bracket the hopes and disappointments of the field. In *The Modularity of Mind*,[16] Fodor defined the conditions requiring mental activities to be modular and independent of their context. Seventeen years later,[22] he acknowledged that the inescapably subjective nature of psychological activities, shown by the empirical dependence upon context, had compelled him to abandon the model of a rational, computer-like brain. Fodor's progression to a very different point of view is symptomatic of a fundamental problem: despite their best efforts, cognitive psychologists have failed to identify modules of mental activity with measurable brain parameters. This is a very strong statement that stands in opposition to the thousands of papers claiming to have localized a mental activity.

COGNITIVE BRAIN ACTIVITY IS NOT LOCALIZED

In addition to the difficulties arising from the effects of context on the practice of modules, fMRI experiments showed that cortical activations during behavior requiring cognition were spread over many brain regions. They were not reproducible across contexts, nor were they uniquely localized, as were the primary responses to sensory inputs, exemplified by the rat whisker discussed above. (Examples of widespread response to the mental concepts are given below.) In using sensory responses as a model for finding brain regions that correspond to modules, cognitive neuroimaging has always been inclined toward a localizationalist view of brain function. Fodor, for example, in his early support of cognitive neuroimaging, contended that Franz Joseph Gall (1758–1828), the advocate of phrenology, "appears to have had an unfairly rotten press."[24] Fodor had not required a strict localization of modules, but to him and many other neuroimagers, the localization of specific cognitive and mental processes seemed the logical way of viewing the organization of the brain. Delocalizationalist views have been adduced by Karl Lashley,[25] among others. By means of careful dissections, he showed that the efficiency of a complex mental function is proportional to the extent of a brain injury within a large area. These views were supported by the Russian neuroscientist A. R. Luria, who described how a given area of the brain can be involved in relatively few or many different behaviors, depending on brain injury and training.[26] The contemporary neurophysiologist E. R. John[27] has pointed out that delocalized concepts of brain function, despite substantial empirical scientific support, have receded from the forefront of neuroscience and been replaced by the localizing powers claimed by cognitive neuroimaging. In Chapter 6 we will continue the discussion of localization in terms of the energy expended in localized and delocalized activities.

THE STRUCTURE OF DIFFERENCING EXPERIMENTS

To present detailed analysis of functional imaging experiments, I turn to two rigorous criteria that originally defined modularity in cognitive neuroscience as offered by Ed Smith, a much-respected Cognitive Neuroscientist.[28] For a differencing experiment to ascribe a cognitive modular process to a unique brain region, he felt it was necessary that:

   (a) A cognitive modular process P, embedded in different tasks or
        contexts, always maps to the same brain region.
   (b) A brain region supporting a specific modular process, P, responds
        uniquely to that process.

As experimental formulations of the basic assumptions of Cognitive Neuroscience, these twin criteria reflected the requirements that different cognitive processes, such as memory or attention, were separable (or modular) and their brain responses were uniquely localized and therefore also modular. If supported by imaging results, they lead to the conclusion that activation of a specific brain region is necessary and sufficient for the specific mental process to take place. If, and only if, the data show modularity of both cognitive processes and brain localizations, then cognitive neuroscience can provide an objective model of how the brain supports cognition. In this case, the brain will have been shown to function locally in response to input modules that have been properly identified by cognitive psychology. In other words, if mental processes are modular, they will have been explained physically by brain activities, thus freeing us from the uncertainties of subjective reports.

WILLED ACTION: AN ILLUSTRATIVE
IMAGING EXPERIMENT

Many experiments show the paradox created by interpretations that test the strict criteria of cognitive neuroscience. The first example examines the experimental test of whether an experiment satisfies the criterion (a) that a process P always maps to the same brain region. This example will show that the meaning of "the same brain region" depends on how narrowly or broadly a "localized" region is defined. Our early fMRI experiments[29] reproduced an earlier PET[30] experiment that studied "willed action," in which novel tasks, presumed to embody this mental activity, were contrasted with routine tasks during verbal or sensorimotor stimulations where "willed action" was missing. The novel verbal task—to generate words beginning with a specific letter—tested verbal fluency, while the routine, or control, task was to repeat a word. Analogously, the novel sensorimotor task was to move either of two fingers when one was touched, while the routine task required that the subject move only the finger being touched. The differences between the tasks were taken to reflect *internal* "willed action" as opposed to *external* response determination.

The difference maps between the novel and routine tasks for both modalities found activations in the dorsolateral prefrontal cortex (DLPFC) and provided detailed coordinates for the centers of activation. In the verbal task, the differences located the activation in the left DLPFC and the anterior cingulate, whereas the sensorimotor coordinates were bilaterally located in the DLPFC and the anterior cingulate. Chris Frith and his colleagues identified a common volume of PET activation in the DLPFC, which they assigned to the common "willed action" component in the different tasks. From this they concluded that "an association between response generation (willed action) and activity in DLPFC has been consistently observed in different PET studies."[30]

However, although our later fMRI data[29] replicating the PET study gave the same results as the PET experiment and confirmed that both verbal and sensorimotor difference images showed activation in the DLPFC, they also provided unambiguous evidence that the two modalities activate significantly different regions of the DLPFC. The fMRI motor and verbal localizations in the left DLPFC are 21 mm apart—a clear separation of responses to the two modalities—while the verbal task shows no response in the right DLPFC, although the motor task does show such a response. Examination of the PET results showed identical locations to the fMRI results: in both experiments, the strong left-hemisphere response to the verbal tasks contrasted with the bilateral response to motor tasks, which clearly distinguished the two modalities! In other words, although the fMRI and PET results were identical, the two reports came to different conclusions. The PET authors, who were theoretically predisposed to accept modularity of both the psychological activities that they called "willed action" and the brain responses, which they measured, concluded that a broadly defined "DLPFC" was activated by "willed action" expressed by tasks in both modalities. The fMRI conclusion,[29] by contrast, emphasized the different experimental locations of verbal and motor activations, although both are to be found in the large brain volume that the PET workers characterized as the DLPFC.[30]

The PET interpretation resorts to an alternative, less focused description of a brain region (i.e., DLPFC) that includes both localizations; instead of using the different brain locations actually activated in the two tasks, it is a common procedure in functional imaging studies to increase the area until a single term will include the data, thereby preserving the appearance of modularity. This process is called canonical correlation analysis.[31] It appeals to Cognitive Neuroscientists because it preserves the nomenclature of identical responses that would support the claim of modularity. To the extent that correlation analysis disavowed hopes of modularity it might serve as the beginnings of an empirical psychology. Far from being an isolated example, the procedure I have described is a common instance of present-day interpretations of functional imaging results, in which large brain areas (e.g., the prefrontal cortex or the precuneus amygdala) are assigned to subjective concepts (of executive function or of default activity, respectively). In this light, large brain areas can be seen as an approximate, empirical description of mental activities. As with verbal descriptions, they offer pragmatic descriptions of brain activities but neither the reproducibility nor the precision required by the strict form of Cognitive Neuroscience, yet they are often referred to in those rigorous terms.

FMRI STUDIES OF WORKING MEMORY

Part (b) of Smith's criteria for modularity, that a region be activated by only one modular process, is routinely not satisfied by results. An example is found in our early papers on working memory.[32,33] Working, or short-term, memory is a commonly defined cognitive activity that has been extensively studied by fMRI. It describes the kind of memory utilized, for example, to retain a telephone number that one has looked up in a directory during the few seconds it takes to pick up the telephone. The distinction between working memory (WM) and long-term memory (LTM) goes back at least as far as William James, who argued that they were qualitatively different.

Over the past 15 years, thousands of functional imaging studies of WM have been carried out in an attempt to identify unique linkages between brain regions and mental processes. At the beginning of 2011, PubMed listed 23,805 references to WM, of which 2,782 acknowledge the use of neuroimaging. In our typical fMRI experiment, the control images, which required attention but not memory, were subtracted from the images of the memory task.[33] The difference image showed an activation of the right prefrontal cortex. However, when the degree of attention demanded in the control condition was increased,[32] the difference signal decreased. Therefore, attention and working memory, as defined by these simple tasks, overlapped in neuronal activation. In short, the experiment could claim that a specific brain activation served WM only by disregarding the finding that a task requiring only attention activated the same localized region as the WM task.

These typical early experimental results did not support the model of a computer-like brain processing modular cognitive representations that are uniquely localized to exclusive brain modules, as demanded by Smith's criteria (a) and (b) above.

POSSIBLE CORRECTIVES TO SIMPLE DIFFERENCING

Ed Smith responded to criticism of the rigorous model proposed for WM by Cognitive Neuroscience.[28] He acknowledged that the simple-subtraction method was circular and open to the criticism that attention and WM activate the same brain region. In a laudable scientific attempt to strengthen the validity of the method, Smith acknowledged that finding an image upon subtraction did not prove its origin and proposed "two kinds of correctives to the simple-subtraction strategy." One was to "study relatively primitive or non-decomposable cognitive processes" to explain the overlap of WM and attention. The other was to use "converging evidence" for this purpose.

Smith's first corrective addressed the requirement that the activation by WM of a brain region must be unique. He accepted that "attention" activated the same region as WM. He further acknowledged that many fMRI results showed that tasks not involving a process P can activate the same region as P. Smith resolved this failing of modularity by emphasizing that when WM is broken into components, the activity of attention is found to be a property of WM. The similar neural response to attention and WM, he claimed, was a consequence of attention being a component of WM. Thus, he concluded that the finding "is evidence *for* the concept of WM, not *against* it" (emphasis added). To preserve the modularity of brain responses, it had been necessary for Smith to sacrifice the separateness or modularity of two highly prized concepts of cognitive psychology, "attention" and "working memory," by proposing that these concepts overlap. However, it is self-contradictory to claim that the fMRI results support the uniqueness of brain modularity while at the same stroke discarding the orthogonality of cognitive modules whose distinctiveness forms a traditional basis of Cognitive Neuroscience.

In his second corrective, Smith hypothesized that when a process activates a particular area, a lesion of that area must inhibit any task involving the process. Lesions had provided an early physiological basis for distinguishing between WM and LTM. However, in 2008, a review article by Smith's long-time colleague John Jonides and his associates assessed the validity of the lesion criteria for identifying cognitive processes involved in WM.[34] They noted that studies of brain-injured patients who showed a deficit in WM but not in LTM "or vice versa from lesion(s)" had implied that WM and LTM are separate systems. However, "a meta-analysis comparing regions activated during verbal LTM and WM tasks indicated a great deal of overlap." From an analysis of imaging data, Jonides and his coauthors concluded that WM and LTM "are not architecturally separable systems—at least not in the strong sense of distinct underlying neural systems. Instead the evidence points to a model in which short-term memories consist of temporary activations of long-term representations." After more than a decade of intensive research, it seems that imaging studies do not support a neuronal distinction between WM and LTM. Moreover, the value of lesions as converging evidence was called into question by the authors, who showed that lesion localizations did not coincide with the fMRI assignments of WM and LTM brain areas.

I want to emphasize that I am not making any judgment about what empirical localizations and correlations of brain activities with behavior can be found or are held by experimentalists. I am only saying that the deductive results predicted by the computer-like brain model proposed by the original framework of Cognitive Neuroscience described in the early literature by Smith, Posner and Raichle, and many others, are not found experimentally.

EMPIRICAL NATURE OF WORKING MEMORY

Although fMRI data are still being interpreted as though these rigorous standards have been met, Smith and Jonides seem to have accepted the necessity of a limited empiricism, whereby the performance of WM is broken into components that are defined so as to fit the imaging results. The need to subdivide psychological concepts into components was recognized early in WM studies, when Baddeley, soon after proposing WM, broke it down into discrete mental acts.[35] In accepting this breakdown, modern students of WM have from the beginning abandoned Fodor's standards for a logical, computer-like brain activity in the interest of seeking an empirical understanding based on fMRI studies. In an effort to fit the imaging data, Jonides and colleagues describe

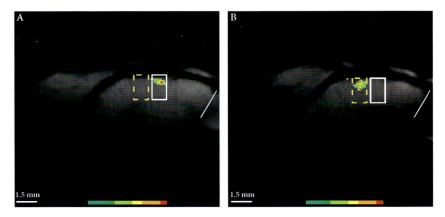

Figure 5.1 An fMRI experiment with D1 and D4 whisker stimulation showing highly localized activation in two contiguous slices.

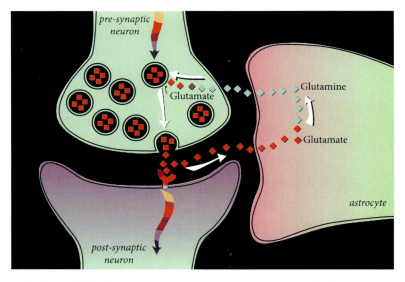

Figure 6.1 A model of glutamate–glutamine neurotransmitter cycling between neurons and astrocytes.

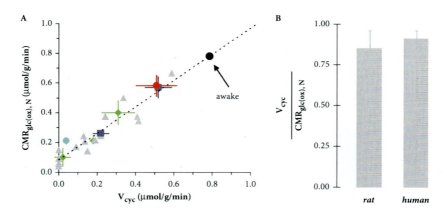

Figure 6.2 ^{13}C MRS and PET results of baseline energy.

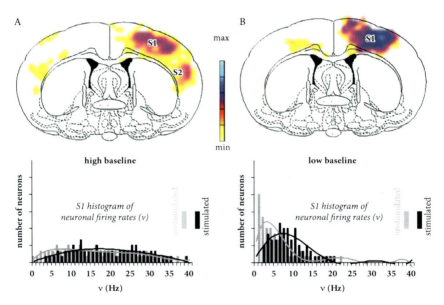

Figure 6.3 Averaged fMRI maps (from two rats, two single runs, 30-s block design, forepaw stimulation) of anterior coronal slices under halothane showed weak widespread activities beyond contralateral primary (S1) and secondary (S2) somatosensory cortices (**A**), whereas under α-chloralose they showed strong localized activation in contralateral S1 (**B**).

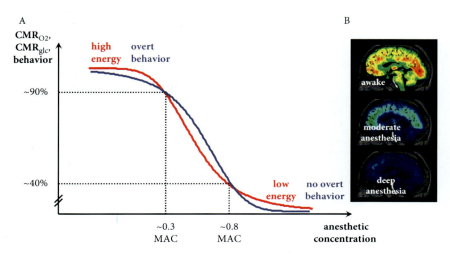

Figure 7.1 (**A**) Loss of consciousness with anesthesia, as assessed by behavioral output and cerebral energy as measured by PET. (**B**) PET energies at different states of anesthesia. Hot colors indicate higher energy demand.

several psychological components of WM that have been proposed. These components arise from decomposing WM into encoding, maintenance, and rehearsal, shifts of attention, and retrieval, some of which are classified as executive functions. In addition, separate buffers in the brain are proposed to support different forms of information (verbal, object, and spatial information are located in separate regions), as well as activated regions attributed to capacity, interference, and storage, and episodic buffers that increase the importance of long-term semantics.

A meta-analysis by Wager and Smith[36] showed that large brain areas are activated by WM and assigned them to Brodmann's areas by using a set of WM component processes similar to that used by Jonides and colleagues. Twenty-four possible combinations of materials and executive functions form the parameter space into which the imaging results of the PET and fMRI studies of WM were assigned. The meta-analysis showed that, even when limited to the three parameters of the type of material being remembered (verbal, object, and spatial), the activations were distributed in 22 Brodmann's areas widely spread throughout a large fraction of the cerebral cortex. With 72 (24×3) variables, the significance of $p < 0.05$ achieved in a half-dozen of the assignments of component activations to brain regions is not very meaningful. The results do not find a brain region characteristic of WM; rather, they find, of the many possible regions, several that (with limited significance) are claimed to respond to a component psychological activity. These conclusions of widespread activations are similar to results by Jonides and colleagues and show that a meta-analysis of essentially all existing data does not improve the identification of brain modules that Jonides and colleagues found in a specific experiment. But the components of a task—for example, the way the data have to be updated—are the context in which the memory is expressed. The context of the WM task—that is, whether it is presented as words or shapes, whether or not they require manipulation, or executive functions, or one of the many other proposed components—overwhelms any uniqueness proposed for brain localization of WM. As Fodor has shown, when the results depend upon "context," the logical structure of brain function is lost and the theory and experiments must be considered as components of an empirical science.

Any attempt to describe the present state of the field would be too ambitious, but a few speculations about the future value of these data might be in order. A growing sophistication is apparent in which the breakdown of the concept of WM into components is becoming acceptable, thereby implicitly acknowledging that there is no single module of WM but many brain components. Instead, empirical relations between components are investigated. For example, Roth and Courtney[37] compare the images obtained when WM is updated with information from sensory stimulation or from long-term memory. Their results, they suggest, identify a single fronto-parietal network that is active when updating WM, regardless of the source of the information.

EMPIRICAL STUDIES OF REPRESENTATIONS

Even though it is a much-contested position, as shown above, the loss of modularity is a widely held position that was pointed out directly and very early by Karl Friston and his colleagues as "the trouble with cognitive subtraction."[38] In this paper and others at the same time, these investigators proposed that different data-processing methods could possibly produce modular brain responses by including interaction terms or higher-order correction to the GLM used to interpret data such as now are being realized in canonical correlation analysis. These proposals to produce modularity suggested that the representations being used for the mental processes underlying the behavior were valid but that complicated nonlinear brain responses caused the apparent loss of a modular brain response. Much later,[39] Friston suggested that modularity could perhaps be improved by using network representations of the brain processes instead of the representations of cognitive psychology. These proposals open large areas of experimentation, which, until explored, allow one to maintain a belief in the possibility of a computer-like brain handling complex stimuli.

WORKING MEMORY AS AN EXAMPLE
OF GENERAL BRAIN ACTIVITY

It is becoming increasingly apparent that the brain activations associated with WM are among the general brain activities used in cognitive processes. Other meta-analyses showed a similar lack of a unique localization for other functions identified by cognitive psychology, such as different forms of memory or attention. In an extended meta-analysis of functional imaging results, Cabeza and Nygard identified widespread locations from a variety of cognitive parameters in the different brain regions.[40] However, "in keeping with the goal of the review," they emphasized consistencies in the responses, concluding that "specific brain regions are consistently activated by specific cognitive challenges" and that "some brain regions are activated by several different cognitive demands." It must be noted, however, that by "brain regions" Cabeza and Nygard mean about 30 Brodmann's areas in which activations of WM, perception, attention, episodic memory, and procedural memory are found. The broad locations assigned to these functions by these findings are similar to the WM results discussed above and show how widespread are the activations introduced by cognitive tasks.

It is necessary to emphasize this shift from the earlier rigorous model to the present loosely defined experimental consensus because imaging research is being extended to localize ever-more-elaborate modules postulated for mental processes, on the assumption that objective understanding has been obtained. In an extreme case, "objective" neuroimaging of social concepts now threatens to replace traditional social science research. For instance, prominent scientific journals, even the *New York Times*, have published results that claim cerebral localizations of political judgments made by Democratic and Republican voters.[41] Images showing greater prefrontal activity among Democrats have been interpreted as evidence that their votes are more rational (rationality being a loose empirical attribute of the prefrontal brain region). Republicans, on the other hand, are reported to have shown higher activations of the amygdala, which is attributed to more emotional processing.

Studies like this one have been mocked as phrenological fMRI, a term whose accuracy becomes clear when one recalls that as long ago as 1836, Orson Squire Fowler and Lorenzo Fowler reported to have localized and measured the degree of "republicanism" in the brain from bumps on the scalp.[42] Similar extensions of differencing fMRI experiments to the courtroom claim support from the modularity postulated by cognitive neuroscience, a claim that extensive experimentation has so far failed to justify.[43] Furthermore, in applications of fMRI experiments to the social sciences, common claims of high statistical probabilities have been shown to suffer from a methodological error.[44] The full significance of this conclusion is still not widely acknowledged in the field, so that social sciences are tantalized by claims of objective brain location of concepts.

EVIDENCE AGAINST COMPUTER THEORIES OF MIND

The last years of the twentieth century were a troubled time for Cognitive Neuroscience. In addition to the unsupportive imaging results, NMR studies of brain energetics and neuronal activity revealed inconsistencies within the computer theory of mind assumed by Cognitive Neuroscience. The assumption of a computer-like brain that would be turned on by cognitive stimuli was confounded by results showing that the fMRI BOLD signals observed in certain brain regions were consistently negative during stimulation.[45] By the time these negative BOLD signals became noteworthy, the role of cerebral energetics and metabolism in brain function was well developed,[46] and knowledge in these areas was advancing rapidly. Looking ahead to the next chapter, where these advances are described in detail, combined ^{13}C MRS, electrophysiology, and fMRI results provided an easy explanation of negative BOLD signals. These studies showed that the changes of energy measured in a typical cognitive task, obtained from the calibrated fMRI signal,[47] amounted to at most a few percent of the total energy consumption, obtained from interpretation of ^{13}C MRS data.[48] Both incremental and total energies were used to support functional processes triggered by neuronal firing, such as ion pumping and glutamate neurotransmitter release. Energy supported neuronal activity of both the baseline state (in the absence of external stimulation) and the increments (during stimulation), while the baseline energies were much larger.

It had long been known that the resting brain consumed a great deal of energy, but that usage had been considered distinct from the functional usage by neuronal firing because of an erroneous analysis of energy usage.[49] However, once ^{13}C MRS results showed that nearly all the brain energy supported activities associated with neuronal firing,[50] the high baseline energy could no longer be regarded as nonfunctional. Hence, the underlying, but rarely expressed, assumption of the computer theory of mind—that the brain was active only in response to a sensory or cognitive input, and remained inactive in the absence of the need to process information—was contradicted by the decreases in energy from the baseline level, reported by negative BOLD signals. These signals had implied a decrease in energy below zero, a description that made no sense. The implications of these neurophysiological results for brain functioning are discussed in the next chapter on neuroenergetics.

NOTES

1. Roy & Sherrington (1890). On the regulation of the blood-supply of the brain *J. Physiol. London, 11*, 85–108.
2. Siesjo, B. (1978). *Brain energy metabolism.* New York: Wiley.
3. Mosso, A., as reported in James, W. (1890). *Principles of psychology.* New York: Dover Press.
4. For a review, see Sokoloff, L. (2004). Energy metabolism in neural tissues in vivo at rest and in functionally altered states. In R. G. Shulman & D. L. Rothman (Eds.), *Brain energetics and neuronal activity* (pp. 11–31). Chichester: John Wiley.
5. Sokoloff, L. (1981). Localization of functional activity in the central nervous system by measurement of glucose utilization with radioactive deoxyglucose. *J. Cereb. Blood Flow Metab., 1*(1), 7–36.
6. Reivich, M., Kuhl, D., Wolf, A., Greenberg, J., Phelps, M., Ido, T., Casella, V., Fowler, J., Hoffman, E., Alavi, A., Som, P. & Sokoloff, L. (1979). The [^{18}F] fluorodeoxyglucose method for the measurement of local cerebral glucose utilization in man. *Circ. Res., 44*, 127–137.
7. Phelps, M. E., Huang, S. C., Hoffman, E. J., Selin, C., Sokoloff, L. & Kuhl, D. E. (1979). Tomographic measurement of local cerebral glucose metabolic rate in humans with (F-18)2-fluoro-2-deoxy-D-glucose: validation of method. *Ann. Neurol, 6*, 371–388.

8. Kwong, K. K., Belliveau, J. W., Chesler, D. A., Goldberg, I. E., Weiskoff, R. M., Poncelet, B. P., Kennedy, D. N., Hoppel, B. E., Cohen, M. S., Turner, R., Cheng, H. M., Brady, T. J., & Rosen, B. R. (1992). Dynamic magnetic resonance imaging of human brain activity during primary sensory stimulation. *Proceedings of the National Academy of Sciences USA, 89*, 5675–5679.

9. Ogawa, S., Tank, D. W., Menon, R., Ellerman, J. M., Kim, S. G., Merkle, H., & Ugurbil, K. (1992). Intrinsic signal changes accompanying sensory stimulation: functional brain mapping with magnetic resonance imaging. *Proceedings of the National Academy of Sciences USA, 89*, 5951–5955.

10. Blamire, A. M., Ogawa, S., Ugurbil, K., Rothman, D. L., McCarthy, G., Ellerman, J. M., Hyder, F., Rattner, Z., & Shulman, R. G. (1992). Dynamic mapping of the human visual cortex by high-speed magnetic resonance imaging. *Proceedings of the National Academy of Sciences USA, 89*, 11069–11073.

11. Bandettini, P. A., Wong, E. C., Hinks, R. S., Tikofsky, R. S., & Hyde, J. S. (1992). Time course EPI of human brain function during task activation. *Magn. Reson. Med., 25*, 390–397.

12. Ugurbil, K., Adriany, G., Andersen, P., Wei, C., Gruetter, R., Hu, X., Merkle, H., Kim, D. S., Kim, S. G., Strupp, J., Hong, X., & Ogawa, S. (2000). Magnetic resonance studies of brain function and neurochemistry. *Ann Rev. Biomed. Eng., 2*, 633–660.

13. Yang, X., Hyder, F., & Shulman, R. G. (1997). Functional MRI BOLD signal coincides with electrical activity in the rat whisker barrels. *Magn. Reson. Med., 38*, 874–877.

14. Bartels, A., & Zeki, S. (2005). The chronoarchitecture of the cerebral cortex. *Phil. Trans. R. Soc. London B Biol. Sci., 360*(1456), 733–750.

15. Hubel, D. H. (1988). *Eye, brain, and vision.* New York: Scientific American Library.

16. Fodor, J. (1983). *The modularity of mind.* Cambridge, MA: Bradford Books, MIT Press.

17. Posner, M. I., & Raichle, M. E. (1994). *Images of mind.* New York: Scientific American Press.

18. Ibid. (p. 23).

19. Ward, N. S., & Frackowiak, R. S. (2004). Towards a new mapping of brain cortex function. *Cerebrovasc. Dis., 17*(Suppl 3), 35–38.

20. Wittgenstein, L. (1953). *Philosophical investigations.* Oxford: Blackwell Press.

21. Nichols, M. J., & Newsome, W. T. (1999). The neurobiology of cognition. *Nature, 402*, C35–C38; Erratum in *Nature* (2000), *403*(6769), 575.

22. Fodor, J. (2000). *The mind doesn't work that way.* Cambridge, MA: MIT Press.

23. Ibid. (p. 25).

24. Op cit., Fodor (1983) (p. 14).

25. Lashley, K. (1951). *Cerebral mechanisms in behavior* (pp. 112–136). New York: Wiley.

26. Luria, A. R. (1966). *Higher cortical functions in man.* New York: Harper & Row.

27. John, E. R. (2006). The sometimes pernicious role of theory in science. *Int. J. Psychophysiol., 62*(3), 377–383.

28. Smith, E. E. (1997). Research strategies for functional neuroimaging: A comment on the interview with R. G. Shulman. *J. Cogn. Neurosci., 9*(1), 167–169.

29. Hyder, F., Phelphs, E. A., Wiggins, C. J., Labar, K. S., & Shulman, R. G. (1997). Willed action: a functional MRI study of the human prefrontal cortex during

a sensorimotor task. *Proceedings of the National Academy of Sciences USA,* *94,* 6989–6994.

30. Frith, C. D., Friston, K., Liddle, P. E., & Frackowiack, R. S. J. (1991). Willed action and the prefrontal cortex in man: a study with PET. *Proc. Roy. Soc. Lond. B, 244,* 241–246.

31. Cordes, D., Jin, M., Curran, T., & Nandy. R. (2012). Optimizing the performance of local canonical correlation analysis in fMRI using spatial constraints. *Hum. Brain Mapping, 33*(11), 2611–2626.

32. Shulman, R. G. (1996). Interview with Robert G. Shulman. *J. Cogn. Neurosci., 8*(5), 474–480.

33. McCarthy, G., Blamire, A. M., Rothman, D. L., Gruetter, R., & Shulman R. G. (1993). Echo-planar magnetic resonance imaging studies of frontal cortex activation during word generation in humans. *Proceedings of the National Academy of Sciences USA, 90,* 4952–4956.

34. Jonides, J., Lewis, R. L., Nee, D. E., Lustig, C. A., Berman, M. G., & Moore, K. S. (2008). The mind and brain of short-term memory. *Ann. Rev. Psychol., 59,* 193–224.

35. Baddeley, A. (1986). *Working memory.* Oxford, UK: Oxford Univ Press.

36. Wager, T. D., & Smith, E. E. (2003). Neuroimaging studies of working memory: a meta-analysis. *Cogn. Affect. Behav. Neurosci., 3,* 255–274.

37. Roth, J. K., & Courtney, S. M. (2007). Neural system for updating object working memory from different sources: sensory stimuli or long-term memory. *Neuroimage, 38,* 617–673.

38. Friston, K. J., Price C. J., Fletcher P., Moore C., Frackowiak, R. S., & Dolan, R. J. (1996). The trouble with cognitive subtraction. *Neuroimage, 4,* 97–104.

39. Friston, K. J. (2009). Modalities, modes, and models in functional neuroimaging. *Science, 326*(5951), 399–403.

40. Cabeza, R., & Nyberg, L. (2000). Imaging cognition II: An empirical review of 275 PET and fMRI studies. *J. Cogn. Neurosci., 12*(1), 1–47.

41. Kaplan, J. T., Freedman, J., & Iacoboni, M. (2007). Us versus them: Political attitudes and party affiliation influence neural response to faces of presidential candidates. *Neuropsychologia, 345,* 55–64.

42. Fowler, O. S., & Fowler, L. N. (1836). *Fowler's practical phrenology, giving a precise elementary view of phrenology* (62nd ed.). New York: Fowler & Wells.

43. Patel, P., Meltzer, C. C., Mayberg, H. S., & Levine, K. (2007). The role of imaging in United States courtrooms. *Neuroimaging Clinics of North America, 17,* 557–567.

44. Vul, E., Harris C., Winkielman, P., & Pashler, H. (2009). Puzzlingly high correlations in fMRI studies of emotion, personality, and social cognition. *Perspectives on Psychological Science, 4,* 274–290. These authors criticized a common statistical procedure in applying fMRI to the social sciences. Basically, results with high significance were obtained by measuring the responses of a population to a stimulus and then repeating the experiment on the same population, assuming they were a representative sample.

45. Shulman, G. L., Corbetta, M., Buckner, R. L., Raichle, M. E., Fiez, J. A., Miezin F. M., & Petersen S. E. (1997). Top-down modulation of early sensory cortex. *Cereb. Cortex, 7*(3), 193–206.

46. Rothman, D. L., Sibson, N. R., Hyder, F., Shen, J., Behar, K. L., & Shulman, R. G. (1999). In vivo nuclear magnetic resonance spectroscopy studies of the relationship between the glutamate-glutamine neurotransmitter cycle and functional neuroenergetics. *Phil. Trans. R. Soc. Lond. B, 354*, 1165–1177.

47. Kida, I., Kennan, R. P., Rothman, D. L., Behar, K. L., & Hyder, F. (2000). High-resolution CMR(O2) mapping in rat cortex: a multiparametric approach to calibration of BOLD image contrast at 7 Tesla. *J. Cereb. Blood Flow Metab., 20*(5), 847–860.

48. Shulman, R. G., & Rothman, D. L. (1998). Interpreting functional imaging studies in terms of neurotransmitter cycling. *Proceedings of the National Academy of Sciences USA, 95*, 11993–11998.

49. Creutzfeldt,O. (1975). Neurophysiological correlates of different functional states of the brain. In D. H. Ingvard & N. A. Lassen (Eds.), *Alfred Benzon Symposium VII* (pp. 21–46). New York: Academic Press.

50. Sibson, N. R., Dhankhar, A., Mason, G. F., Behar, K. L., Rothman, D. L., & Shulman, R. G. (1997). In vivo ^{13}C NMR measurements of cerebral glutamine synthesis as evidence for glutamate-glutamine cycling. *Proceedings of the National Academy of Sciences USA, 94*, 2699–2704.

6

Brain Energy and the Work of

Neurotransmission

---

aving reviewed philosophies and scientific methods available for brain research, I turn to the experimental bottom-up approach to brain function, primarily focusing on developments made with my colleagues during the past 20 years. The strength of bottom-up studies—experiments that propose and test hypotheses that are consistent with the data and the laws of physics—is their capacity to develop physical understanding. However, this strength also gives rise—almost immediately—to the question of how helpful they can be in studying the higher-level questions of brain function. I will suggest that, as our understanding grows, new concepts and, more importantly, new questions emerge with an immediacy that previous understanding could neither visualize nor answer. We shall turn to these questions after discussing the neurophysiological advances made at the level of energetics and metabolism by noninvasive imaging techniques.

The studies follow the great physiologists of the nineteenth century, Herman von Helmholtz and Claude Bernard, who created systemic physiology by the application of classical physics and chemistry to *in vivo* chemical reactions centered on the generation and usages of energy. The rates of metabolic pathways serving the physiological needs of the body have long provided the understanding of normal systemic function. The developments of systemic physiology, continuous since their time, have been strengthened by the ability of noninvasive brain measurements of metabolic fluxes to integrate energy and rates of neurotransmission. Noninvasive NMR methods have opened a new window on neurophysiology that is consolidating our understanding of the control and energetics of neuronal firing.

Our neurophysiological studies start by measuring the chemical generation of brain energy simultaneously with measuring the flux of neural transmitters released and cycled during neural firing—a unique cerebral metabolic pathway.

Physiology has long been the starting point for detailed molecular and physical descriptions of normal functions that rely on the fundamental physical parameters of energy and work. There is no need to burrow down further into the quantum level once we reach an understanding in the classical terms provided by thermodynamics. The experiments to be described have the degree of explanation afforded by quantitative measurements of the rates of chemical reactions *in vivo*. How far can we go from these results toward an understanding of the more complex human functions that are the ultimate goal of neuroscience?

Even with the contemporary emphasis on genomics, it is recognized that bodily processes take place at the metabolic level. Neurophysiology becomes doubly important when we realize that in addition to the normal functioning of the brain, it holds the key to the identification and control of neurological diseased states. The parameters that will be discussed in this chapter—glutamate neurotransmitter flux, the accompanying flow of gamma aminobutyric acid (GABA), and the dependence of these rates on the behavioral state—provide insights into normal function and neurological diseases. Our intention is to show how noninvasive measurements of cerebral metabolism, energy, and work have create a reliable starting point for the biophysical exploration of behavior. First, though, before we consider what brain energetics and metabolism can tell us about behavior, we must consider how they can be measured.

NONINVASIVE MEASUREMENTS OF CEREBRAL ENERGY

Neurophysiological properties of brain firing and metabolism can be studied only *in vivo*. Accordingly, recent measurements of brain energy consumption and work have profited from the noninvasive methods of magnetic resonance and PET. Brain energy has been measured in humans and animals by following the rates of glucose oxidation that provide the main energy for the brain, while at the same time following the release of the primary neurotransmitters that are coupled to the rates of neuronal firing. .

Bottom-up studies of cerebral functions start by evaluating the delivery and consumption of glucose and oxygen. The human brain consumes high levels of energy, which are obtained almost exclusively from the oxidation of glucose, as reported by Kety and Schmidt in 1948.[1] They determined rates by measuring the concentration of metabolites flowing into the brain, in the arterial blood, and flowing out in the venous blood. They established the high rates of glucose and energy consumption and found that glucose was almost the exclusive substrate of brain metabolism. Under normal healthy conditions the brain produced equal amounts of CO_2 for each mole of O_2 consumed, while the O_2 consumption was approximately six times the consumption of glucose, all as expected from the complete oxidation of glucose. By the 1970s it was clear that to a first approximation brain energy came from the complete oxidation of glucose, and this energy was being consumed in the resting state by the brain at a higher rate than in the average body tissue. The results showed a marked reduction in global energy production from diabetic acidosis, moderate hypoglycemia, and during lower levels of consciousness from surgical levels of anesthesia, as well as from coma and cerebral ischemia.

Local measurements by Louis Sokoloff[2] of the uptake of 2-deoxyglucose (2DG) (which is phosphorylated but not subsequently oxidized) enabled local measurements of CMR_{glc} to be made in animals. Extensions of the 2DG method (using a fluorinated analogue) to humans by PET[3] allowed local measurements of CMR_{glc}, which were soon extended to CMR_{O2} and CBF.

¹³C MRS STUDIES OF GLUTAMATE NEUROTRANSMISSION

Although by the 1970s a basic understanding of brain energy production and consumption was in hand, the question remained as to what fraction of brain energy was devoted to neuronal firing—in other words, how efficient was the brain's use of energy? In the 1970s, calculations based on earlier results on the great axon of the squid led to the disconcerting claim that only a small fraction of brain energy was consumed in neuronal firing and signaling.[4] The question of efficiency was resolved in the 1990s by MRS experiments that measured the rates of glucose oxidation and the release of neurotransmitters in the same experiment. Those results, to be described next, showed that nearly all the brain energy was used by the neurons and glia in support of neuronal firing.[5]

¹³C MRS tracks metabolic pathways by labeling substrates or fuel molecules such as glucose by enriching the concentration of an NMR-visible stable isotope, ¹³C, which has a natural abundance of ~1.1%. *In vivo* ¹³C MRS measurements then follow the metabolism of glucose through the appearance of the ¹³C label in metabolite pools down the pathway. Rates of these metabolic pathways are determined by measuring the label appearance as a function of time into pools of metabolites whose total concentrations are known. In 1982, initial studies of pathways in microorganisms and perfused organs by ¹³C MRS were extended to intact animal models and to human limbs.[5] Three years later, the Yale School of Medicine established a Magnetic Resonance Center equipped with superconducting magnets capable of following *in vivo* the fluxes through metabolic pathways in the human torso and brain. Since that time, *in vivo* ¹³C NMR has been applied to study a variety of metabolic pathways and systems in animals and humans in our laboratory and in other laboratories around the world.[6,7]

The brain functions by signaling between neurons. Communication between neurons occurs at the synapses, the junctions of neurons, and their connections with surrounding astrocytes. Cortical communication between neurons is fundamental to the neurobiological view of brain function. Generally, activations are transmitted across the synaptic gap by small molecules acting as neurotransmitters. Neurotransmitters are studied by many methods. New neurotransmitters are continually being discovered, identified, and localized, while their receptors and their release are investigated by genetic and chemical methods. MRS measurements allowed us to consider neurotransmitters as a class of metabolites that are intermediates in pathways whose concentrations and fluxes can be studied *in vivo* as they participate in neurotransmission, one particularly important aspect of metabolism. Their neurochemical pathways serve the brain's primary function of communicating across synapses. Since their rates of release and recognition are an intrinsic part of brain activity, it is to be expected that this neurotransmitter activity would be related to brain energy consumption.

The ^{13}C MRS experiments have focused on just these points—how neurotransmitter fluxes are responsible for neuronal signaling, and how this process depends on brain energy consumption. Among the dozens of neurotransmitters that have been identified and characterized, several (dopamine, serotonin, acetylcholine, and norepinephrine) have been studied intensively for decades. Two neurotransmitters (glutamate and GABA) stand out because of their high concentrations (in the millimolar range). In the mammalian cortex, more than 90% of the neurons serve these two highly concentrated neurotransmitters. Glutamate is excitatory, serving to transmit activation, while GABA, in the minority, serves an inhibitory function.[8] The high concentrations of glutamate and GABA have enabled their high-resolution NMR signals to be observed *in vivo* by ^{13}C MRS. Enriched ^{13}C glucose is particularly useful for following pathways and measuring fluxes by MRS experiments that follow the flow of ^{13}C label into pools of cerebral metabolites. ^{13}C MRS has measured the flow from ^{13}C-enriched glucose to ^{13}C glutamate, which was used to calculate the flux through the tricarboxylic acid cycle, an intermediate step on the way to the full oxidation of glucose. CMR_{O2} was calculated from the glucose flux to glutamate. ^{13}C MRS measurements of the label flow from glucose into the glutamate pool are weighted toward neuronal energy consumption, since the large brain glutamate pool is primarily neuronal. The values of CMR_{O2} that were determined by this method in experiments on rats and humans agreed well with the values found in the scientific literature, thereby validating the ^{13}C MRS method of measuring oxygen consumption, and the energy as the oxidation of glucose.

Technical improvements to NMR dependent on larger and stronger magnets have made it possible to measure the label flow from glutamate into glutamine in the human brain in the same experiment that measures the flow of glucose into glutamate. Glutamine, although not a neurotransmitter, had been proposed to be an intermediate in the glutamate neurotransmitter cycle. The ability to follow in time, *in vivo*, the label flow into glutamate, and subsequently into glutamine by ^{13}C MRS, opened glutamate neurotransmitter cycling and the coupled cerebral energy production to quantitation. The cycle was originally proposed in the 1970s from ^{14}C and ^{15}N studies of extracts and slices of rat brains.[9] Additional support came from studies localizing specific enzymes in neurons and astrocytes. However, when we started these experiments, the importance of this pathway *in vivo* had not been accepted because of conflicting evidence about their magnitude from studies of brain slices and other *in vitro* preparations.

Figure 6.1 shows the modern version of the cycle as provided by the ^{13}C MRS results.[10] Glutamate stored in vesicles in the presynaptic neuron is released into the synaptic cleft by firing in response to neuronal depolarization. Once

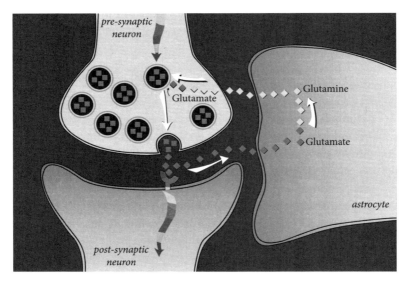

Figure 6.1 A model of glutamate–glutamine neurotransmitter cycling between neurons and astrocytes. The rate of the glutamate-to-glutamine cycle (V_{cyc}) has been quantitated by ^{13}C MRS. Action potentials or spikes (shown by *black arrows*) reach the presynaptic terminal to initiate the release of vesicular glutamate into the synaptic cleft. This activates the glutamate receptors in the postsynaptic neuron, which is a step required in the propagation of spiking activity to the adjacent neuron (in an all-or-none manner). The extracellular glutamate is removed rapidly by Na^+-coupled transport into astrocytes, where it is converted into glutamine. The synthesized glutamine then passively diffuses back to the neuron, and after reconversion to glutamate, is repackaged into vesicles. *Note*: see color insert.

(Reproduced with permission from Shulman, R. G., & Rothman, D. L. (1998). Interpreting functional imaging studies in terms of neurotransmitter cycling. *Proceedings of the National Academy of Sciences USA, 95*, 11993–11998.)

released, it diffuses across the gap until it is recognized by a glutamate receptor on the postsynaptic surface, which triggers the subsequent postsynaptic potential changes that send the signal on to the next neurons. The released glutamates diffuse to the membranes of the surrounding glia, into which they are co-transported down the Na$^+$ gradient. The glial enzyme, glutamine synthetase, then converts glutamate to glutamine, thus consuming one ATP and one NH$_3$. Glutamine is transported across the glial membrane, through the intracellular space, and into the neuron, where an enzyme reconverts it to glutamate. Finally, the glutamate is repackaged into vesicles, where it is ready to restart the cycle.

The first ^{13}C MRS experiments established that the flux from glutamate to glutamine was far from negligible.[6] It was, in fact, comparable to the rate of glucose oxidation, indicating that the glutamate/glutamine cycle is a major metabolic pathway in the brain. Subsequent studies showed that the rate of neuronal glucose oxidation increases with the rate of the glutamate/glutamine cycling.[10] This finding indicated that brain energy metabolism is coupled directly to glutamate neurotransmission and therefore to brain function.

GLUTAMATE CYCLING AND NEURONAL ENERGY CONSUMPTION

Soon after the first promising observation of ^{13}C flows in human brains, a comprehensive study extended these results to the rat brain and reached quantitative conclusions in the more easily manipulated animal model. It established that the cycling model was equally valid in rat and human brains and that the rates of cycling and glucose oxidation are similarly coupled in both species. The rates of oxidation and cycling were studied over a wide range of brain activities in the rat, taking the animals from deep anesthesia, with no neuronal firing, through lighter states of anesthesia, to a lightly anesthetized state in which neuronal firing was enhanced by seizures. Simultaneous measurements of the ^{13}C flow into glutamate determined the cerebral metabolic rate of glucose oxidation (CMR$_{glucose(ox)}$), and the subsequent flow into glutamine determined V$_{cycle}$, the glutamate neurotransmitter cycling rate. The cycling flux (V$_{cycle}$) plotted in Figure 6.2A against energy consumption (CMR$_{glucose(ox)}$), which was determined from the measured rates of glucose oxidation, was fitted very well with a straight line of

$$CMR_{glucose(ox)} = V_{cycle} + 0.10 \qquad [1]$$

all in the same units of micromoles/g.min.[10]

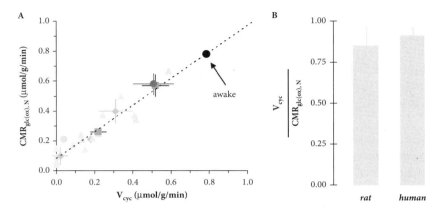

Figure 6.2 ^{13}C MRS and PET results of baseline energy. (**A**) Experimental results of the rates of neurotransmitter cycling (V_{cyc}) and of the metabolic rate of neuronal glucose oxidation (CMR$_{glc(ox),N}$). Values for the rat brain reported between 1998 and 2006 are assigned to original sources in Shulman et al. (2009). (**B**) The ratio of neurotransmitter cycling to neuronal glucose oxidation in the nonanesthetized resting awake states in rat and human brain. *Note*: see color insert.

(Reproduced with permission from Shulman, R. G., Hyder, F., & Rothman, D. L. (2009). Baseline brain energy supports the state of consciousness. *Proceedings of the National Academy of Sciences USA, 106*, 11096–11101.)

This plot is significant in several respects. First, it establishes a quantitative molecular relationship between cortical oxidative energy production and the glutamate neurotransmitter flux, a measurement that is related to neuronal firing. Second, it provides the rate of glucose oxidation, which is a convenient measurement of this activity. A third significant finding can be seen from the value of CMR$_{glucose(ox)}$ at the intercept in Figure 6.2A where V_{cycle} falls to zero. This corresponds to the state of flat EEG where neuronal firing has ceased and was brought about by deep pentobarbital anesthesia. At this point, glucose oxidation had fallen to about 15% of the value in the awake nonanesthetized state. Only this small fraction of the basal, resting cerebral energy consumption is needed to support the brain in the absence of spike activity, thereby indicating that in the awake, resting basal state, about 85% of the energy consumption supports neuronal firing and its concomitant neurotransmitter flux. The large fraction of brain energy consumption dedicated to cycling in the rat is similar to results in the resting awake human (Fig.6.2B).This high level of brain neurotransmitter activity in the absence of specific stimulations was a novel finding that required a fundamental reevaluation of the results obtained from higher-level brain studies, including those dependent on functional imaging.

Another unexpected feature of the data seen in Figure 6.2A, where the cycling flux (V_{cycle}) is plotted against the rate of neuronal glucose oxidation

(CMR$_{glucose(ox)}$), is the slope of unity. This value means that, for every additional glucose molecule oxidized in a neuron, one glutamate is released as a neurotransmitter and cycles through glutamine. The stoichiometry allows changes in neurotransmitter flux (which can be measured directly in this sort of ^{13}C NMR experiment) to be derived from measured changes in oxygen consumption.

These MRS results have answered the questions Creutzfeldt[4] raised in his calculations of brain energy usage based upon the squid axon. In the resting, awake mammalian brain, nearly all of the energy is consumed in processes that are coupled to synaptic activity. These results, it must be emphasized, do not show that this energy is consumed in the glutamate/glutamine cycling pathway; that process is but one step in the energy-consuming reactions that are tightly coupled to neuronal firing. Efforts to apportion the energy to the different steps—that is, the re-pumping of ion gradients in the presynaptic and postsynaptic neurons, the resting potential, and other minor energy-consuming steps—have supported the observation that the rate of glutamate/glutamine cycling is directly proportional to the rate of neuronal firing.[11] These calculations of an "energy budget" have, to within their accuracy, supported the idea that the energy consumption is tightly coupled to the neuronal firing. However, definitive support for the efficient use of energy by the processes coupled to neuronal firing is shown by the 1:1 relationship between the metabolic fluxes of glutamate to glutamine for neurotransmission and of glucose oxidation. These results are being explored by molecular and cellular models, seeking a molecular mechanism for the stoichiometric coupling of glutamate neurotransmission and glucose oxidation.[12]

CALIBRATION OF FMRI ENERGETICS

MRI experiments locate and measure the concentration of water molecules in space, thereby generating an image. However, the BOLD fMRI method provides additional information by responding to the concentration of deoxygenated hemoglobin in the red blood cells.[13] It does this by acquiring imaging data in such a way that the intensity of the image decreases with the concentration of this paramagnetic deoxygenated form of hemoglobin. The binding of oxygen to hemoglobin is an equilibrium process, so that the fraction of hemoglobin that is bound to oxygen increases with the concentration of oxygen. Therefore, the BOLD signal intensity reflects the change in oxygen concentration during the stimulus being tested.

The BOLD signal is related to metabolism since the oxygen concentration increases with increases in the rates of the cerebral metabolic rate of oxygen consumption (ΔCMR$_{O2}$) and the cerebral blood flow (ΔCBF). (Increases in the rate of oxygen consumption by stimulation, which might lead one to expect a decrease in oxygen levels, are overcompensated by larger increases in blood flow, which bring in arterial blood with a high level of oxygen.) Results show that CBF increases about four times as much as CMR_{O2} during activation in response to a sensory stimulation, and since the flow brings in heavily oxygenated arterial blood, it causes the concentration of oxygen to increase in the activated voxel. Analysis of the fMRI signal allows the value of CMR_{O2} to be determined from the data, providing that ΔCBF is measured independently.[14] This is readily done by alternative MRI techniques, so that fMRI BOLD signals can be converted into measures of energy metabolism. BOLD results that have been quantitated this way so as to yield incremental energies are referred to as "calibrated BOLD."[14] In this way, fMRI can make valuable measurements of the same metabolic parameters as MRS. The fMRI determinations complement the MRS evaluation of total CMR_{O2} because they measure differences of these values (ΔCMR_{O2}) between two conditions with high spatial and temporal resolution. The combined applications of these MRS and calibrated BOLD methods in the human or animal brain can provide a brain map of the total and incremental rates of energy consumption under a wide variety of circumstances. When the quantitative values of total energy from ^{13}C MRS and of incremental energy (ΔCMR_{O2}) from BOLD were available, the point was made[15,16] that the incremental energies were only a small fraction of the total, a result whose significance is discussed below.

CORRELATION OF METABOLIC AND ELECTRICAL ENERGIES

The electrical nature of neuronal activity has been the mainstream of brain studies since Luigi Galvani's findings at the end of the eighteenth century. In subsequent studies, brain activity, which has the ability to process information and mediate behavior, has been expressed as the coordinated electrical activity of neurons. Although chemical aspects of neuronal activity are well recognized, the electrical properties of neuronal firing and action potentials still constitute, for the traditional neurophysiologist, the gold standard for understanding brain function. Neurophysiological studies of energy and metabolism starting with Sherrington, and culminating in their noninvasive determinations described above, have until recently played an ancillary role in brain function, which for many neuroscientists continues to be defined as the electrical activities of synapses. For metabolism and energetics to play a significant role in neuroscience, they had to be related to the electrical activity of coordinated neuronal systems. In other words, the work performed by the electrical activities of ensembles of neurons, which supports brain functions, must be quantitatively related to the energy consumption of the same region. The connection between energy consumption and neurotransmitter release, a direct consequence of neuronal firing, was established by the ^{13}C MRS experiments described above. However, a direct correlation of energy consumption and firing rates would cement the relationship and allow direct connections between different experimental results.

The convergence between these apparently different levels of observation—between the firing of ensembles of neurons in the volume element set by fMRI, and the energetics and metabolism in that volume—has been established by studies of the work done and energy expended by the system of neurons.[17-19] Neuronal work will be proportional to the neuronal firing rates, which can be measured in a representative ensemble containing several hundred neurons and presented as a histogram plotting the number of neurons firing at each frequency. The energy expended by a spiking neuron to perform the work associated with firing (the chemical work required for neurotransmitter release and cycling and for pumping ions across membranes) is assumed to be the same for each firing and therefore to be linear with the firing rate. By multiplying the number of neurons firing at any frequency by their firing rate, the relative energy consumption (CMR_{O2}) for the neuronal ensemble can be related to the work of neuronal firing by summing over the population

$$CMR_{O2} = G \sum_i N_i v_i \qquad [2]$$

where the running index i spans the entire range of frequencies in the histogram; N_i is the number of cells firing at the frequency v_i in the ensemble; and G is a scaling factor that connects neuronal density and metabolic rate per neuron with the number of neurons in a volume whose energy is measured.

Present research continues to extend the quantitative relation between neuronal activity and chemical energy consumption. If the *same* neuronal population is measured across different states (i.e., if N_i does not change across states of the subject), then changes in CMR_{O2} are proportional to shifts in firing rates within the neuronal ensemble. In rat brains, changes in CMR_{O2} between different activation states, measured by fMRI, agreed with relative changes in CMR_{O2} calculated by Equation 2 from multi-unit electrode measurements of neuronal firing rates in a representative neuronal ensemble.[18,19] Furthermore, the total CMR_{O2} measured by ^{13}C MRS at different states of activation, achieved by different levels of anesthesia in rats, was proportional to the total firing rates of a representative ensemble.

In summary, this energetic consensus finds that the lion's share of the energy consumed by the brain is produced by the oxidation of glucose and is devoted to the work required by the electrical activity of neurons. The correlation between neuronal firing rates and their energy consumption relates the energy consumption in voxels to firing rates of representative ensembles of neurons by expressing both as CMR_{O_2}. The energetic relationship between metabolic measurements of neurotransmission and glucose oxidation and the electrical measurements of neuronal firing rate quantitatively establishes the equivalence of both approaches to electrochemical brain activity. With this equivalence established, the relative magnitude and importance of these different measurements can be fruitfully compared, whereas previously they were limited to separate, incommensurable reports of the same phenomenon.

EFFECTS OF BASELINE ENERGY ON FMRI

In addition to the traditional neuroimaging approach of varying the stimulus input, the brain's endogenous total energy can also be modified and serve as an independent variable. The magnitude and spreading of the fMRI signal are two observable properties that have been shown to depend on the total energy.

I first consider the dependence of the amplitude of the stimulated signal on the total brain energy.[19-21] Studies have used different values of total activity at controlled external conditions (e.g., dark vs. light) or internal (e.g., sleepy vs. alert) to evaluate the effects of baseline energy on the response to stimulation.[18,19] In a rat study, for example, the same sensory stimulation was applied at two different resting-state levels, where CMR_{O_2} differed by about 30%, created by different anesthetic doses.[18] Different amplitudes of fMRI activations in the contralateral primary somatosensory cortex were detected in the two states. The BOLD response was significantly stronger in the low-energy baseline state (i.e., high anesthetic dose) compared to the high-energy state (i.e., low anesthetic dose) (Fig. 6.3). In similar stimulations of the cat O^{17} MRS measurements showed that the magnitude of the evoked response upon stimulation is larger from the lower level of baseline activity.[22]

Human experiments need strategies to manipulate the baseline activity level without affecting subsequent evoked responses. An elegant study by Paisly and colleagues[23] used a novel stimulus paradigm to alter the baseline energy in the visual cortex of the awake human. They measured the BOLD signal, the CBF, and the CMR_{O_2} during stimulation in two conditions. One was the normal resting condition and the other was a lower baseline created by a continuous negative stimulus. During stimulation there was a larger metabolic response from the lower state so that both conditions reached the same metabolic state. The authors concluded that "the negative response is a functionally significant index of neural deactivation." As in the anesthetized rat, this study reported an

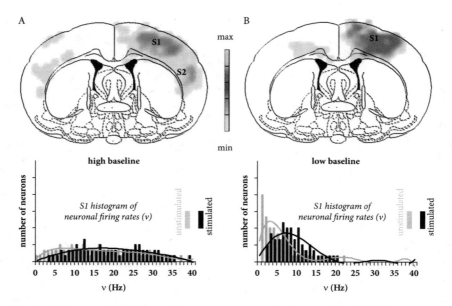

Figure 6.3 Averaged fMRI maps (from two rats, two single runs, 30-s block design, forepaw stimulation) of anterior coronal slices under halothane showed weak widespread activities beyond contralateral primary (S1) and secondary (S2) somatosensory cortices (**A**), whereas under α-chloralose they showed strong localized activation in contralateral S1 (**B**).

Total activity in the two states represented in the two histograms by distribution of firing rates (10-s bins) in the primary somatosensory ensemble of 200 neurons for halothane (**A**) and α-chloralose states (**B**). Activity under halothane is dominated by the rapidly signaling neuronal subgroup, which seems unaffected by stimulation. The slowly signaling neuronal subgroup, shifting to higher frequencies on stimulation, is more responsive under α-chloralose. [Copyright 2007 by The National Academy of Sciences of the USA.] *Note*: see color insert.

(Modified from. Maandag, N. J. G., Coman, D., Sanganahalli, B. G., Herman, P., Smith, A. J., Blumenfeld, H., Shulman, R. G., & Hyder, F. (2007). Energetics of neuronal signaling and fMRI activity. *Proceedings of the National Academy of Sciences USA, 104*(51), 20546–20551.)

inverse relationship of the magnitude of the response with the baseline energy that in the awake, human visual cortex reached the same activated energy state regardless of the baseline. This quantitative assignment of energy to the negative signal completed the work of Shmuel and colleagues,[24] who had shown that neuronal activity is responsible for the major component of the negative response.

The baseline energy level also significantly affects the spread of the fMRI evoked response. These effects are seen in the fMRI studies in rats at the two anesthetic states, characterized by very different baseline energies, whose fMRI amplitudes were discussed in the previous paragraph.[19] Forepaw stimulation

was administered in both states to excite the contralateral primary somatosensory cortex. At high baseline there were activations in anterior brain
regions (Fig. 6.3A), which included primary and secondary contralateral
somatosensory cortices, and in posterior areas (not shown) there were activations in secondary areas of visual and auditory cortices, and in the thalamus
and perirhinal cortex. At low baseline, however, strong activations were confined to the contralateral somatosensory cortex, with insignificant activities
elsewhere (Fig. 6.3B).

The neuronal firing rates were represented in histograms to depict each state
in the presence and absence of stimulation. Neuronal histograms in the two
states allowed the populations to be divided into subgroups of slow signaling
neurons and rapid signaling neurons,SSN and RSN respectively, with firing rates
less than or greater than 20 Hz. The most conspicuous difference between the
two anesthetized states of different energy was the dominance of RSN activity
under halothane Fig. 6.3A in contrast to the α-chloralose condition(Fig.6.3B).
At the high baseline energy, a majority (80%) of total energy is used for RSN
activity, whereas at low baseline, the SSN activity accounts for more than half
(60–70%) of total energy consumption.). The RSN population correlated with
the greater delocalization of BOLD activations (Fig. 6.3A). At high baseline
energy, with greater RSN activity, widespread activations were observed, while
at low baseline energy, strong activations were confined to the contralateral primary somatosensory cortex.

Similar consequences of anesthesia have been reported in humans, where
light anesthesia eliminated responses of higher-order regions and limited the
fMRI signals to the sensory cortex.[25–29] A human fMRI study by Sperling and
colleagues showed that activations became more localized upon sedation.[25] The
high baseline state was the normal awake condition, whereas the low baseline
state was achieved with lorazepam—a benzodiazepine agonist that lowers CMR_{glc}
by about 30% from the awake level.[26] The stimulus was a cognitive paradigm of
face and name associations. Similar to the anesthetized fMRI rat study, this
awake human fMRI study[27,28] showed a greater spread of activation at the
higher baseline energies. The dependence of the degree of delocalization of the
fMRI signal on the baseline energy may have relevance for recent fMRI studies
on coma patients, which show, in some cases, highly active sensory cortices
during tasks, whereas the higher-order regions, active for those stimuli in the
awake state, are inactive in all the patients.[29] A simultaneous evaluation of the
baseline energy by PET with the fMRI response could help distinguish whether
the sensory response was supported by the recovery of specific pathways or by
the more general delocalized activity from higher baselines.

These experiments have related the results of fMRI measurements reflecting
the energy consumption of a voxel, with sub-millimeter dimensions, to the

energy consumption of the microscopic neurons. Our hypothesis that the RSN activity supports intracortical signaling, and that it mediates communication between the activated sensory unit and distal cortical areas, is based on the correlation between high RSN activity in the activated somatosensory cortex and widespread BOLD activations. The experimental relations between macroscopic properties of brain activity and microscopic neuronal activity has allowed us to propose a separation of neuronal activity into subpopulations on the basis of firing rates that has implications for understanding the relationships between local processing within sensory units and global activity patterns of neural ensembles.[30] This connection between the microscopic (electrophysiology) and the macroscopic (neuroimaging), an empirical identification of two subpopulations, suggests that we can move slightly, but with some degree of assurance, within the total neuronal population toward the important but distant complexity of heterogeneous activities of individual neurons.[31]

BASELINE ENERGIES INFLUENCE PSYCHOLOGIES

The high rate of neuronal activity in the unstimulated awake state, shown by the ^{13}CMRS experiments, was inconsistent with the implicit assumption of the computer-like brain postulated by Cognitive Neuroscience, which made no allowance for energy consumption in the absence of stimulation. Under that model, specific brain regions, shown by positive BOLD or PET signals, when activated were considered to have used brain energy to perform a task. A reduction in brain energy from its value at rest would be inconsistent with the computer-like brain whose energy expenditure was acknowledged only during stimulation. This inconsistency was brought home by the reproducible observations of negative BOLD signals in 1997.[32] Although negative signals showing a regional decrease in energy consumption created no problem for the high baseline energies reported by ^{13}CMRS,[15] they were not consistent with a computer-like brain.

Gusnard and Raichle[33] moved away from a computer-like brain, noting that there was a common region of negative BOLD signals during a wide range of tasks—for example, visual and auditory attention, language processing, memory and motor activity—that were well known to create positive signals in other brain regions. The consistency with which the posterior cingulate cortex and adjacent precuneus showed these decreases led them to suggest that there might be an organized mode of brain function, which, they hypothesized, is associated with the representation (monitoring) of the world around us.[34] They defined this region (including similar decreases in the dorsal medial prefrontal cortex) as a default mode, whose activity would be continuously available and not curtailed until attention was shifted elsewhere by the focused needs of a task. It must be emphasized that the default mode was defined by the incremental BOLD activity (negative) during goal-directed actions, an activity that represents only a few percent of the total energy.

As the neurophysiological results accumulated, Gusnard and Raichle proposed that the brain had a "baseline" state in which the activities of the default regions were assigned to a broad range of psychological functions, centering on self-awareness or self-attention. Their claim that a baseline level of energy exists has been confusing since the identification of a baseline state, originally described by the negative BOLD signal, representing a few percent decrease of the total energy, has drifted in their subsequent publications to where it is sometimes considered to be the total energy, described as "the energy consumed by this ever active messaging, known as the brain's default mode, is about twenty times that used by the brain when it responds consciously to a pesky fly or another outside stimulus."[35]

The properties postulated for the default mode were augmented when synchronous oscillations at low frequency (0.1–0.01 Hz) of the unstimulated BOLD signal, originally reported by Biswal and Hyde,[36] were found to be characteristic of this region.[37] Greicius and colleagues showed that these low-frequency BOLD signals were synchronous between regions of the default mode. Raichle then proposed that a large-scale network organization of the default mode was revealed by these patterns of spatial coherence in the spontaneous fluctuations of the resting BOLD signal. This interpretation, depending on a signal that represents only a few percent of the total energy or activity, has been enthusiastically received by the neuroimaging community as a network of psychologically assigned correlations.

However, it is clear from this discussion that the properties of the proposed default mode are similar to previously characterized psychologically assigned positive fMRI increments of the same large brain areas. The difference is that now it is being implied, in the face of the actual negative incremental BOLD data, that the large total or intrinsic activity has been assigned to these psychological activities. This empirical effort to understand precuneus and prefrontal activities would be strengthened by distinguishing between the two measurable kinds of brain activity, the high level of total brain energy and the smaller incremental brain energies measured in response to stimuli. In the next chapters we show how physiological measurements of the total and incremental energies can be separately related to observable behaviors without resorting to psychological assumptions that weaken the reliable correlations of brain activities and observable behavior.

NOTES

1. Kety, S. S., & Schmidt, C.F. (1948). The effects of altered arterial tensions of carbon dioxide and oxygen on cerebral blood flow and cerebral oxygen consumption of normal young men. *J. Clin. Invest.*, 27(4), 484–492.

2. Sokoloff, L. (2004). Energy metabolism in neural tissues in vivo at rest and in functionally altered states. In R. G. Shulman & D. L. Rothman (Eds.), *Brain energetics & neuronal activity*. Chichester: John Wiley & Sons.

3. Sokoloff, L., Reivich, M., Kennedy, C., Des Rosiers, M. H., Patlak, C. S., Pettigrew, K. D., Sakurada, O., & Shinohara, M. (1977). The [^{14}C] deoxyglucose method for the measurement of local cerebral glucose utilization: theory, procedure, and normal values in the conscious and anesthetized albino rat. *J. Neurochem.*, 28(5), 897–916.

4. Creutzfeldt, O. D. (1975). Neurophysiological correlates of different functional states of the brain. In *Alfred Benzon Symposium* VII. New York: Academic Press.

5. For a comprehensive review of the determination of brain energetics and their relation to brain function, see Shulman, R. G., & Rothman, D. L. (2004). *Brain energetics & neuronal activity: Applications to fMRI and medicine.* Chichester: John Wiley & Sons.

6. Sibson, N. R., Dhankhar, A., Mason, G. F., Rothman, D. L., Behar, K. L., & Shulman, R. G. (1998). Stoichiometric coupling of brain glucose metabolism and glutamatergic neuronal activity. *Proceedings of the National Academy of Sciences, USA*, 95(1), 316–321.

7. Shulman, R. G., Hyder, F., & Rothman, D. L. (2002). Biophysical basis of brain activity: Implications for neuroimaging. *Q. Rev. Biophys.*, 35:287–325.

8. Deutch, A. Y., & Roth, R. H. (1999). Neurotransmitters. In M. J. Zigmond, F. E. Bloom, C.I. Story, J. L. Roberts, & L. R. Squire (Eds.), *Fundamental neuroscience* (pp. 193–234). New York: Academic Press.

9. Van Den Berg, C. J., & Garfinkel, D. (1971). A stimulation study of brain compartments. Metabolism of glutamate and related substances in mouse brain. *Biochem. J.*, 123, 211–218.

10. Hyder, F., Patel, A. B., Gjedde, A., Rothman, D. L., Behar, K. L., & Shulman, R. G. (2006). Neuronal-glial glucose oxidation and glutamatergic-GABAergic function. *J Cereb. Blood Flow Metab*, 26, 865–877.

11. Atwell, D., & Laughlan, S. B. (2001). An energy budget for signaling in the grey matter of the brain. *J. Cereb. Blood Flow Metab*, 21, 1133–1145.

12. Magistretti, P. J., Pellerin, L., Rothman, D. L., & Shulman, R. G. (1999). Perspective: Neuroscience "energy on demand." *Science*, 283, 496–497.

13. Ogawa, S., Menon, R. S., Tank, D. W., Kim, S. G., Merkle, H., Ellerman, J. M., & Ugurbil, K. (1993). Functional brain mapping by blood oxygenation level-dependent contrast magnetic resonance imaging. A comparison of signal characteristics with a biophysical model. *Biophys. J.*, 64, 803–812.

14. Kida, I., & Hyder, F. (2006). Physiology of functional magnetic resonance imaging: energetics and function. *Methods Mol. Med.*, 124, 175–195.

15. Shulman, R. G., & Rothman, D. L. (1998). Interpreting functional imaging studies in terms of neurotransmitter cycling. *Proceedings of the National Academy of Sciences USA*, 95, 11993–11998.

16. Hyder, F., Rothman, D. L., & Shulman, R. G. (2002). Total neuroenergetics support localized brain activity: Implications for the interpretation of fMRI. *Proceedings of the National Academy of Sciences USA*, *99*, 10771–10776.

17. Raichle, M. (1998). Behind the scenes of functional brain imaging: a historical and physiological perspective. *Proceedings of the National Academy of Sciences USA*, *95*(3), 765–772.

18. Smith, A. J, Blumenfeld, H., Behar, K. L., Rothman, D. L., Shulman, R. G., & Hyder, F. (2002). Cerebral energetics and spiking rates: The neurophysiological basis of fMRI. *Proceedings of the National Academy of Sciences USA*, *99*, 10765–10770.

19. Maandag, N. J., Coman, D., Sanganahalli, B. G., Herman, P., Smith, A. J., Blumenfeld, H., Shulman, R. G., & Hyder, F. (2007). Energetics of neuronal signaling and fMRI activity. *Proceedings of the National Academy of Sciences USA*, *104*(51), 20546–20551.

20. Li, A., Gong, L., & Xu, F. (2011). Brain-state-independent neural representation of peripheral stimulation in rat olfactory bulb. *Proceedings of the National Academy of Sciences USA*, *108*, 5087–5092.

21. van Eijsden, P., Hyder, F., Rothman, D. L., & Shulman, R. G. (2009). Neurophysiology of functional imaging. *Neuroimage*, *45*(4), 1047–1054.

22. Zhu, X. H., Zhang, N., Zhang, Y., Uğurbil, K., & Chen, W. (2009). New insights into central roles of cerebral oxygen metabolism in the resting and stimulus-evoked brain. *J. Cereb. Blood Flow Metab.*, 29, 10–18.

23. Pasley, B. N., Inglis, B. A., & Freeman, R. D. (2007). Analysis of oxygen metabolism implies a neural origin for the negative BOLD response in human visual cortex. *Neuroimage*, 36, 269–276.

24. Shmuel, A., Augath, M., Oeltermann, A., & Logothetis, N. K. (2006). Negative functional MRI response ccorrelates with decreases in neuronal activity in monkey visual area V1. *Nat. Neurosci.*, 9, 569–577.

25. Sperling, R., Greve, D., Dale, A, Killiany, R., Holmes, J., Rosas, H. D., Cocchiarella, A., Firth, P., Rosen, B., Lake, S., Lange, N., Routledge, C., & Albert, M. (2002). Functional MRI detection of pharmacologically induced memory impairment. *Proceedings of the National Academy of Sciences USA*, *99*, 455–460.

26. Volkow, N. D., Wang, G. J., Overall, J. E., Hitzemann, R. J., Fowler, J. S., Pappas, N., Frecska, E., & Netusil, N. (1998). Regional brain metabolism response to lorazepam in alcoholics during early and late alcohol detoxification. *Alcoholism, Clinical and Experimental Research*, *21*, 1278–1284.

27. Heinke, W., Fiebach, C. J., Schwarzbauer, C., Meyer, M., Olthoff, D., & Alter, K. (2004). Sequential effects of propofol on functional brain activation induced by auditory language processing: an event-related functional magnetic resonance imaging study. *Br. J. Anaesth.*, 92, 641–650.

28. Dueck, M. H. Petzke, F., Gerbershagen, H. J., Paul, M., Hesselmann, V., Girnus, R., Krug, B., Sorger, B., Goebel, R., Lehrke, R., Sturm, V., & Boerner, U. (2005). Propofol attenuates responses of the auditory cortex to acoustic stimulation in a dose-dependent manner: a fMRI study. *Acta Anaesthesiologica Scandinavica*, *49*, 784–791.

29. Davis, M. H., Coleman, M. R., Absalom, A. R., Rodd, J. M., Johnsrude, I. S., Matta, B. F., Owen, A. M., & Menon, D. K. (2007). Dissociating speech perception and

comprehension at reduced levels of awareness. *Proceedings of the National Academy of Sciences USA, 104,* 16032–16037.

30. Buzsaki, G. (2006). *Rhythms of the brain.* New York: Oxford University Press.
31. Adrian, E. D. (1941). Afferent discharges to the cerebral cortex from peripheral sense organs. *J. Physiol., 100,* 159–191.
32. Shulman, G. L., Fiez, J. A., Corbetta, M., Buckner, R. L., Miezin, F. M., Raichle, M. E., & Petersen, S. E. (1997). Common blood flow changes across visual tasks: II. Decreases in cerebral cortex. *J. Cogn. Neurosci., 9*(5), 648–663.
33. Gusnard, D. A., & Raichle, M. E. (2001). Searching for a baseline: functional imaging and the resting human brain. *Nature Review Neuroscience, 2*(10), 685–694.
34. Raichle, M. E., MacLeod, A. M., Snyder, A. Z., Powers, W. J., Gusnard, D. A., & Shulman, G. L. (2001). A default mode of brain function. *Proceedings of the National Academy of Sciences USA, 98*(2), 676–682.
35. Raichle, M. (2001). The brain's dark energy. *Scientific American, 302*(3), 44–49.
36. Biswal, B., Yetkin, F. Z., Haughton, V. M., & Hyde, J. S. (1995). Functional connectivity in the motor cortex of resting human brain using echo-planar MRI. *Magn. Reson. Med., 34*(4), 537–541.
37. Greicius, M. D., Kiviniemi, V., Tervonen, O., Vainionpaa, V., Alahuhta, S., Reiss, A. L., & Menon, V. (2008). Persistent default-mode network connectivity during light sedation. *Hum. Brain Mapp., 29*(7), 839–847.

7

Global Brain Energy Supports the
State of Consciousness

——————

A central question of neuroscience focuses on the role played by brain activities in observable behavior. Studies of consciousness frame this question for brain scientists. The pragmatic analysis and experimental brain energies developed in the previous chapters provide a strategy for studying the neuronal mechanisms that allow a person to exhibit the behavior defining consciousness. Three characteristics of this approach to consciousness, defined and illustrated in this chapter, guide our study into empirical, realizable directions. First, aspects of consciousness are to be defined by a person's observable behavior. Second, these features are to be correlated with and illuminated by neuronal mechanisms that are necessary for their performance but are not sufficient to explain them. Third, the behaviors identifying consciousness are not to be conceptualized and reduced to activities at the level of mental processes. The underlying epistemological basis of these assumptions is that fundamental laws such as those capable of explaining the motion of a frictionless billiard ball or of planetary bodies, long the ideal in physical science, are not the appropriate goal in biological sciences. Rather, behavioral phenomena, once identified, are to be explained by finding mechanisms and properties that are necessary for their occurrence. Proponents of the philosophy of mechanism[1] have shown by historical examples that this kind of understanding has been the normative goal of biological research. For example, once glycolysis had been identified as the transformation of glucose into lactate by yeast, an understanding of the process was reached by the evaluations of the enzymes and intermediates of the pathway, while our understanding of a disease like diabetes or of a sensory perception like hearing is similarly created by identifying its necessary properties or mechanisms. For a biophysicist, the most valuable properties and mechanisms will be found by physical and chemical studies. Essentially, this process depends upon observable identification of the biological phenomenon followed by physical-chemical studies of the properties and mechanisms responsible for its occurrence. In this chapter a person being in the state of consciousness is defined by observations of his behavior; once identified, its properties are elucidated by physical-chemical studies of brain activities. I believe that the state of consciousness can be defined empirically, and understanding how this is done leads us down a path of what can judiciously be said next. However, before we embark upon the turbulent waters exploring behavioral activities by the actions of an organ like the brain, let us examine the more tranquil journey exploring how we understand the role of skeletal muscle in human activities, where the risk of slipping into deductive epistemologies—the tendency to assert what we "know" by appeal to non-experimental data—is less tempting.

ENERGY AND BEHAVIOR

Energy and work have provided a physical basis for understanding the body's functions. The physical work of skeletal muscle and the heart depends on the energy consumed. Muscle energy production during work, which equals energy consumption, is measured by the oxidation of a carbon fuel, mainly glucose, just as it is for the brain. The amount of energy consumed by the arm muscle is equivalent to the work performed by the arm in lifting a specific weight a certain height. In everyday speech, this leads us to say that the muscle performs that work—that the muscle lifts that weight. However, to consider what is really meant by the statement "the muscle lifts the weight," consider the role of the arm muscle during a more complex human task like the groom lifting his bride over the threshold. Recognizing what is actually being done there, we say that the groom lifts the bride and that his muscle supports his effort, or is necessary for him to do so, or that the muscle expenditure of energy to create a force explains his ability to do that work. In other words, physiology has flourished by explaining how the work of the body parts supports observable human functions. It is immediately apparent in this case that other factors, like the groom's intention, the tradition of marriage in our society, and the very existence of a house and threshold, are needed for this activity to occur and that, while the muscle effort is one of the necessary factors, it is not the only one. Physiology does not propose that the muscle work is sufficient to accomplish the human function, merely that it is necessary. Saying that an organ did a certain work, actually performed by the person, is shorthand for saying that the work of the organ supports the human in that effort.

To say that the muscle lifts the bride across the threshold makes no sense and is not intended, yet a similar phrase is often used to explain the support offered by the brain for human functions. Although this elision is innocuous when analyzing muscle work, it leads to serious errors in neurophysiology by assuming that the brain performs an act that should more accurately be attributed to the person. This way of talking has led some neuroscientists to claim that the brain performs mental processes presumed to underlie behavior, whereas all we can observe is the human behavior. Chapter 5 summarizes the common position that brain activity causes a person's action rather than being a supporting factor. (It would not be any more accurate to say that the brain remembered an event, instead conceptualizing it as memory, but in general the conceptualization rather than the performance of the human activity is claimed to be done by the brain.) In place of this assumption, I suggest we should look for the mechanisms by which brain energy is converted to the work of neuronal firing that supports the person's behavior. First, though, we begin with consciousness—before even pondering whether we can say anything useful about consciousness, we must begin by saying what we can about the brain in a conscious person.

THE STATE OF CONSCIOUSNESS: DEFINED BY BEHAVIOR

To understand how brain activity in the form of energy expenditure supports human functions, we must clarify how those functions are defined. Human work, such as remembering, calculating, deciding, or responding, is exemplified in activities that can be identified by behavior: test results show that the person has remembered something, and decisions as to whether remembering has occurred are confidently based upon the person's behavior on the test. However, behavior does not define the mental processes that underlie these activities. They have been the province of academic psychology as well as literature, some philosophies, and lately computer science, economics, and linguistics. For a neuroscientist, behavior provides an observable definition of a phenomenon. When a phenomenon is defined by behavior, it becomes a fact whose mechanisms and properties are suitable subjects for brain research. After behavior is used to decide whether a person is or is not in a state of consciousness, then the brain properties and mechanisms characteristic of that state can be identified and measured. Consciousness is often considered a very difficult problem not only because there are limits in defining it—that is true of all human activities, including remembering and calculating—but because it is often burdened by a wish to define the concept of consciousness in terms of mental activities.

However, if we relinquish that goal and define a person to be in a state of consciousness by his behavior, then brain research can reveal brain mechanisms and properties that support the person in that effort. When a person is in a state defined by observable behavior, the mechanisms by which neuronal activity provides support for the person in that state are opened to neuroscience. Once the muscle was understood to allow the arm to provide a force that the person could apply, physiological research could reveal the mechanisms by which that force was created. The role of the sliding fibers, the consumption of ATP, the metabolism of glycogen and glucose: all could be explained by physical science, and we began to understand muscle function. I propose that defining the state of human consciousness by behavioral indices creates a similar opportunity for neuroscience to study the brain mechanisms supporting the person in that state. As the philosophy of mechanisms[1] has emphasized, understanding consists of surrounding a phenomenon with mechanisms that contribute to its occurrence. For the properties or mechanisms of a phenomenon like consciousness to be unveiled, the existence of particular aspects of consciousness must be identified, distinguished from other forms of consciousness, and ascertained by observable behavior. An understanding of a person in the state of consciousness will now be developed and followed by identifying brain activities necessary for the person to be in that state.

THE STATE OF CONSCIOUSNESS

The model used for our analysis of the brain mechanism supporting human functions, including consciousness, builds upon the work of Maxwell Bennett and Peter Hacker. Bennett and Hacker[2] analyzed and criticized cognitive neuroscientists and their philosophical allies who had assumed that brain activity explained and was responsible for psychological processes manifested by behavior. They showed that it made no sense to ascribe attributes to the brain that only made sense to ascribe to the person. It is the person, they claimed, who remembers something, a statement that can be tested, and it makes no sense to say that the brain remembers, since that statement cannot be distinguished from tests of the person. A brain activity could be necessary for the person's behavior where, for example, an intact, functioning visual cortex was required for the person to see an event, but activity of the visual cortex did not completely explain the person's observable response to a visual scene.

The activities making up consciousness have often been considered as consisting of two forms: Bennett and Hacker called them "intransitive" consciousness and "transitive" consciousness.[3]

In an analogous breakdown Adam Zeman in his comprehensive book[4] "uses parallel definitions of the 'enabling' of and the 'contents' of consciousness" to describe these two aspects of consciousness. Christoph Koch uses the terms[5] "enabling neural correlates of consciousness" and "neural correlates of consciousness." I prefer our terms "state of consciousness" and "acts of consciousness" to describe the two recognizable aspects of consciousness because they include the behavioral definitions that will distinguish these states. In this chapter we investigate the state of consciousness, similar to Bennett and Hacker's intransitive consciousness. This is a condition in which the person is capable of perceiving and interacting with his environment and is sensitive to stimuli. A person may drop out of the state of consciousness "on fainting or being anesthetized and subsequently recover when regaining consciousness."[3] The state of consciousness has no object. It is a matter of being conscious or awake, as opposed to being unconscious or asleep. Bennett and Hacker continue "that there is nothing essentially private about intransitive consciousness. That a person has regained consciousness or is awoken is normally fully visible in his behavior."[6] The state of consciousness is a precondition for any experience. From this definition, a third person's observation can decide that a person either is or is not in that state. I propose that the person being in a state of consciousness is definable by his activities, and the brain can play a role in that state. Assigned this way makes being in that state a reliable fact whose properties and mechanisms can be explored by empirical physical science.

In accordance with the practice in anesthesiology, we have used observations of a person's responses to simple stimuli[7] to define whether or not he is in the state of consciousness: the ability to respond to a stimulus defines the state a person is in but does not define the mental processes that occur during that state. The ability to respond to a stimulus indicates the existence of "the pre-existing organization that determines what factors may be used as stimuli." This quote from Timo Jarvilehto[8] recognizes that the state of consciousness is a property of the person that has been created by his historically continuous interaction with the environment. Organism and environment are separable, but one cannot overemphasize the extent to which the environment has been internalized in forming the person and therefore in determining his response to stimulus. When the anesthesiologist pronounces the patient to be conscious by his ability to answer simple questions, the patient's condition is defined, but this objective measure is also consistent with subjective impressions. An experienced anesthesiologist said to me that in addition to responses to stimuli, "I look into the patient's eyes," meaning that he takes into account the patient's comprehensive interaction with the world. Thus, the person's behavior is not claimed to be a completely objective measure of his state of consciousness, which would have, by a stroke of the pen, simply substituted the behavioral response for the complexities of consciousness, and would have allowed an advanced robot to be defined as in a state of consciousness. Avoiding those possible future quandaries, I see no practical problems in defining a palpable human as being in a state of consciousness by his responses to simple stimuli. The response to simple questions, evaluated by observers as an enabling state, not an unthinking conditioned reaction, gives a **reliable** indication of the patient's effective connection with the world that I call the state of consciousness, whose brain properties can be studied.

The object of study is the person, an entity that includes brain, body, history, and psychological capacities (remembering, perceiving, sensing, etc.) that cooperate to maintain life and homeostasis while interacting with the environment. This definition of the state of consciousness has some overlap with the views of Antonio Damasio, who, as a neurologist and neuroscientist, has written in support of the idea that the study of "mental activity, from its simplest aspects to its most sublime, requires both brain and body."[9] In accepting this neurophysiological account of how body and brain are in continual back-and-forth interactions via chemical and neuronal impulses, I am, at the very least, not assuming that the brain alone is responsible for the person's behavior.

TOTAL GLOBAL ENERGY IS A NECESSARY PROPERTY OF THE STATE OF CONSCIOUSNESS

The hopes of relating brain activity to behavioral states of individuals, such as the state of consciousness, have become possible in recent years by the powers revealed by fMRI, ^{13}CMRS, and PET. Studies like those described in Chapter 6 have been measuring brain energy production, in the form of glucose oxidation, in resting states and during activations in the human or the rat. The most striking result from these experiments is that the total energy consumption supporting neuronal firing is measured by ^{13}MRS and PET and can be distinguished from the incremental energy usually measured by fMRI. The total energy consumption is an order of magnitude larger than the energy changes during stimulation. Nonetheless, most research relating brain activity to behavior has used the smaller fMRI or PET increments (or decrements) to interpret and localize brain activities. To do so was, in effect, to discount the high baseline level of brain activity as irrelevant. It is now possible to consider the total, global brain energy as a valuable parameter of brain activity once it was shown, by ^{13}C MRS as described in Chapter 6, that approximately 80% of this energy is used to support neuronal firing. Until suspicions that a large fraction of this energy was devoted to some nonsignaling purpose, usually called housekeeping, were overcome, the common practice was simply to ignore the large energy. Furthermore, its widespread, delocalized nature also reduced its interest to neuroscientists accustomed to emphasizing the importance of *localized* activities.

Experimental results have allowed us to hypothesize that the total brain energy is a measurable, necessary property of the state of consciousness.

In defining properties of the state of consciousness, I am proposing a functional role for the total brain energy that hitherto has been neglected. PET and MRS experiments showed that a high level of global brain energy consumption was necessary for a person to be in that state. When the high level of brain energy consumption is reduced by anesthesia, sleep, or neuronal pathologies like coma, the person loses the abilities to respond to simple stimuli that had defined his being in the state of consciousness. Limiting parameters to the observables of high global brain energy and the response to simple stimuli explained how the person was defined to be in the state of consciousness with the reliability needed by physical science. For purposes of definition we attend only to the extremes, where a clear-cut answer of "yes" or "no" is possible. The existence of intermediate states where one slips through drowsiness to loss of consciousness does not interfere with the definition of the common extremes.

Since brain energy consumption is a reliable measurement of neuronal activity, this hypothesis correlates total cerebral energetics with reliable observations of behavior. High global brain energies are therefore necessary properties of a person in that state. Our approach finds a functional role for the high-energy baseline activity in the brain. In addition to the high-energy baseline activity other brain activities that are properties of the state of consciousness have been experimentally identified and are discussed below. In this way brain experiments are used to determine a set of neuronal and energetic properties of a person in a behavioral state that enables the person to remember his birthday or to perform simple calculations like addition, which are observable behaviors. Our understanding of brain activities characteristic of the state of consciousness starts with a behavioral identification of the person being in that state and then measures its neuronal properties.

HIGH BASELINE ENERGY AND
NEURONAL ACTIVITY IN THE RAT

Continuous energy supply is imperative for brain function, since endogenous energy reserves are minimal. Normal function needs blood circulation to efficiently provide nutrients and remove waste. The majority of energetic costs for brain work are met by ATP derived from glucose oxidation. To relate brain energy production to brain function, it was necessary to relate the high baseline energy consumption to the firing activity of neurons. Rat experiments were performed using ^{13}C MRS, as detailed in Chapter 6. These results established a quantitative molecular relationship between cortical oxidative energy production and the glutamate neurotransmitter flux that is directly coupled to the rate of neuronal firing. They showed that in the awake, resting state, ~80% of the brain energy consumption was devoted to supporting neuronal signaling.[10] These ^{13}C MRS results, by connecting the energy consumption with the release of glutamate responsible for most of the neurotransmission, showed that the large majority of brain energy consumption is devoted to the work that supports neuronal firing. Direct measurements of the rates of neuronal firing and the rates of glucose oxidation cemented this relationship between energy and neuronal work,[11,12] and typical results confirming that brain energy efficiently supports neuronal firing have been shown in the previous chapter. This equivalence of chemical and electrical approaches to brain work is the basis of converting PET studies of human glucose and oxygen consumption to global brain activity in the resting state and during anesthesia.

ANESTHESIA AND THE ENERGETICS OF CONSCIOUSNESS

In identifying the state of consciousness by the subject's ability to respond to stimuli, we are using criteria established in anesthesiology. Studying brain energies and their changes during the loss of consciousness with anesthesia is an active neurophysiological research area. PET and MRS experiments have measured the energy consumption in brain regions and followed their changes under anesthesia. In the state of consciousness, a person can respond to a stimulus. At deep levels of anesthesia, human subjects are not conscious, as judged from their inability to respond to sensory stimuli and/or questions from the anesthesiologist. While there are many circumstances where humans cannot respond (i.e., sleep, coma, physical impairment, etc.), for the sake of simplicity the definition of unresponsiveness is limited to human individuals who have full expressive faculties. The stipulation that subjects must be able to communicate illustrates that while high brain activity is necessary for a person to be in the state of consciousness, it is not sufficient—the ability to communicate is another necessary property. When consciousness is considered, as in clinical studies, to consist of both aware and awake properties, our measure of responsiveness, where we assume an awake subject, able to perceive and to communicate readily, is a measure of the subject's awareness. (My definition of the state of consciousness, which includes the subject's ability to communicate, creates a practical, observable standard for defining the subject's state. Its clinical usefulness for the pathological locked-in state is discussed below.) In the rat, the conscious state has been identified by the righting reflex, by which the animal always lands on his feet when dropped, an ability that is lost in the deeply anesthetized state. Specific behavioral criteria of the loss of consciousness (i.e., responsiveness in the human and the righting reflex in the rat) have the same dose–response curves for common anesthetics in humans and rats, allowing results from both species to be used in a complementary fashion.[13]

Experiments determining human global energy consumption in the awake state and its reduction under deep anesthesia have been reported by several groups. PET images of brain glucose and oxygen consumption (CMR_{glc} and CMR_{O2}) in varied depths of anesthesia show, to a first order, ubiquitous reduction of brain energy demand from the level of the awake state (Fig. 7.1B).[14-16] All the common anesthetics produce similar global reductions of about 50% in energy consumption at the level suitable for surgery. To a first approximation, these suppressions were not region- or anesthesia-specific, although beyond their first-order similarities small second-order regional differences have been reported.[17] The correlation between the level of global brain energy consumption and the degree of consciousness was the basis of my hypothesis that measurable high global energy is necessary for the person to be in a state of consciousness (Fig. 7.1). (Anesthesia reduces the energy consumption and therefore the firing rate since energy and firing rate are tightly coupled. I have used them interchangeably reflecting the measurement, which in this case is the energy.) The homogeneous reduction in brain energy to anesthetics reported in the groundbreaking PET results by Alkire[14,15] and Kaisti[16] and their colleagues led me to the hypothesis that high homogeneous global energy was a property the person needed to be in the state of consciousness and that its uniform reduction under anesthesia was responsible for the loss of consciousness. In subsequent publications, these authors moved away from this interpretation of their data and suggested that a complex localized set of brain areas was responsible for anesthetic-induced unconsciousness.[17,18] They thus assigned the action of anesthesia to broadly localized, but not global, brain regions by introducing considerations from lesions, functional imaging, clinical observations, default modes, sleep, and so forth. They have suggested that the small differences (of a few percent) in energy reduction by anesthesia in those regions are more causative of the loss of consciousness than is the large global decrease introduced by all anesthetics. At present, the claims of regional specificity do not provide a convincing explanation of the loss of consciousness because the slightly larger reductions do not occur in the same region when the results from different laboratories are compared.[17,18]

The relation between global energies and the loss of consciousness was revealed by comparing measurements at different levels of anesthetics of the

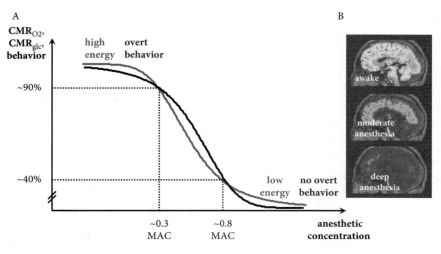

Figure 7.1 (**A**) Loss of consciousness with anesthesia, as assessed by behavioral output
and cerebral energy as measured by PET. (The curves were interpreted by Fahmeed
Hyder from data in Figure 3 from Katoh, T., Bito, H., & Sato, S. (2000). Influence of age
on hypnotic requirement, bispectral index, and 95% spectral edge frequency associated
with sedation induced by sevoflurane. *Anesthesiology, 92*(1), 55–61, and Stullken, E. H.,
Milde, J. H., Michenfelder, J. D., & Tinker, J. H. (1977). The nonlinear responses of
cerebral metabolism to low concentrations of halothane, enflurane, isoflurane, and thio-
pental. *Anesthesiology, 46*, 28–34.) (**B**) PET energies at different states of anesthesia. Hot
colors indicate higher energy demand. *Note*: see color insert.

(Reprinted by permission from Macmillan Publishers Ltd. Alkire, M. T. (2008). Probing the mind:
Anesthesia and neuroimaging. *Clin. Pharmacol. Ther.*, 84, 149–152, copyright 2008.)

global energy consumption by PET and of patient's behavior while being prepared for surgery (Fig. 7.1). The PET images of CMR_{O2} showed the energy consumption in the resting awake state, in an intermediate state, and in the state
of deep anesthesia.[17] Plotting the separate measurements together showed that
the patient's ability to respond to stimuli and the energy consumption both are
sigmoidal with respect to the concentration of anesthetic.[19] The shape of this
response indicates a high degree of correlation of firing between the neurons. If
there were no correlation between neuronal firings, wherein each neuron fired
and used energy independent of all others, the plot of energy consumption
versus concentration of anesthetic would be linear, whereas if neuronal firings
were tightly coupled, the response to deepening anesthesia would be abrupt,
like a phase change. The sigmoidal shape indicates an intermediate degree of
coupling between neurons, providing an insight into neuronal activity supporting the state of consciousness that is unveiled by correlating total energetics and
behavior. While a coupling between the firing of neurons is expected from the
highly credible models of action potential, still the degree of the cooperation

in vivo, a valuable parameter of brain signaling, should be available from these data when refined.

Postulating that global rather than localized energy reductions are responsible for the loss of consciousness is supported by the proposed mechanisms of anesthesia.[13] Three target sites have been identified for the molecular action of all the common anesthetics, and all three sites directly or indirectly inhibit glutamate neurotransmitter activity. Actions of all known anesthetic agents (with the exception of ketamine, which is anomalous in many respects) are consistent with decreases in the glutamate-GABA synaptic activity, which would cause the reductions observed in cerebral energy consumption. Since glutamatergic neurotransmission is widespread throughout the brain, the response to anesthetics (small molecules that diffuse readily throughout the brain) is consistent with the uniform energy reduction observed in the PET experiments. Consciousness is absent during anesthesia when regional energy levels are uniformly reduced by 40% to 50% from the awake resting values. However, the brain does not exist only in either of two extreme states, one conscious and the other not. Rather, existing data (Fig. 7.1) show a continuous variation both of brain activity and of the behavioral properties, from awareness to drowsiness and eventually unawareness as the brain energy level is reduced.

While the fully conscious state can be distinguished clearly from its loss, future experiments might be able to delineate the dependence of detailed behaviors upon these graded transitions. Energy is expected to serve as a unifying parameter in such experiments in that similar behavioral changes could depend upon the global brain energy level that would be reached at different concentrations of the various anesthetics.

ADDITIONAL BRAIN PROPERTIES OF THE STATE OF CONSCIOUSNESS

The high global brain energy measured by PET and ^{13}CMRS in the resting awake state of consciousness has been shown to be a necessary property of this state, judged by the loss of consciousness when the energy is reduced by anesthesia or neurological pathologies. Other brain activities followed by MRI or neuronal electrodes begin to delineate cerebral mechanisms or properties responsible for the phenomenon.

For discussing fMRI experiments, I will follow the conventional usage and describe the total energy in the control state as the "baseline" energy. The baseline energy is compared with the total energy in a subsequent condition when the subject is participating in an experiment. The effects of baseline energies upon fMRI signals were explored in rats at two different baseline energies, as described in Chapter 6. fMRI activations in the two conditions showed very different responses to forepaw stimulations. At high baseline (halothane), there were activations in the somatosensory cortex and several other brain regions. At low baseline, corresponding to a state of deep anesthesia, strong signals were found only in the somatosensory cortex. The comparison of the amplitude and spread of BOLD images of a rat, at the two different levels illustrates how the responses to stimulations are a property of the baseline energy. Several classical neuroimaging studies have agreed with these results, showing that activity patterns from sensory stimuli in anesthetized humans do not extend beyond the sensory cortex.[20] These results suggest that the state of consciousness allows brain-wide responses that do not exist for the animal in deep anesthesia.

The dependence of cerebral energy upon anesthesia has allowed us to correlate behavioral and neuronal properties with energy, some in humans and others in the rat. Additional objective, reliable understandings of what is involved neurophysiologically in producing the state of consciousness can be built gradually from further studies of measurable brain properties. This type of understanding of the state of consciousness, which avoids philosophical and quotidian formulations of consciousness, has the scientific reliability of bottom-up, physically based neurophysiological measurements. The hypotheses that the high brain energy, the widely distributed fMRI signals, and the high multi-unit firings are properties of the global baseline energy could be strengthened if other means, in addition to anesthesia, were available to vary global brain energies or their associated firing rates. An alternative could be to reduce global brain energy by lowering the brain temperature. If the observed properties were truly dependent on total brain energy, as herein proposed, and not on specific mechanisms of anesthesia, then they should change similarly with the energy by lowering brain temperature.

CLINICAL APPLICATIONS

Neuroimaging studies of the consequences of anesthesia have been accompanied by extensive experiments on patients with disorders of consciousness. The terrible consequences of neurological neuropathies have stimulated PET and fMRI studies of patients in an effort to understand the nature of brain activities responsible for these diseases. For diagnostic purposes, consciousness is broken into wakefulness and awareness. Our studies have addressed awareness, where for the purpose of definition we have assumed that the person is awake and able to communicate. With this ability we have defined awareness, or the state of consciousness, by the ability to respond to simple stimuli, and hypothesized that it requires a high level of global brain energy metabolism. In clinical medicine, the loss of consciousness is central in defining and treating persons with disorders of consciousness such as the vegetative state, coma, or locked-in syndrome. Neuroimaging studies of patients with disorders of consciousness have been pursued for diagnosis and treatment that could supplement the rather subjective evaluations upon which the diagnosis depends. These clinical considerations have generated enough enthusiasm for neuroimaging experiments to overcome the experimental difficulties of systematically studying patients and have produced a large body of valuable data. Several groups of dedicated physician researchers in New York; Cambridge, Massachusetts; and Liège, Belgium, have been making these extensive PET measurements of brain energy levels of patients suffering from a loss of consciousness.[21,22] These careful studies, carried out over two decades, have shown that in all but one condition where awareness is lost, brain energy consumption is lowered to about half of the value in normal consciousness, similar to the level observed under deep anesthesia. The results in Figure 7.2 come from homogeneous reductions in brain energy consumption illustrated by the PET results shown in Figure 7.1. Slight increases in brain energy consumption are noted in patients moving between the vegetative state, coma, and minimally conscious states, but therapies trying to increase the energy and to restore consciousness have not been successful. Low brain energies in Figure 7.2, with one exception, invariably accompany the loss of consciousness.

The exception is locked-in syndrome, the horrifying condition in which a person can think and feel with an awareness that can be expressed only by eyelid movements. Once communication has been made possible by the eye blinks, which come from deeper brain regions and bypass the cortex, patients

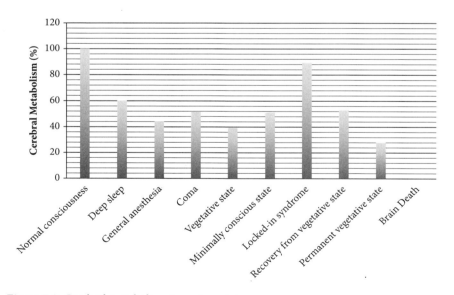

Figure 7.2 Cerebral metabolism in various states.

(From Laureys, S., et al. (2004). *Lancet Neurology, 3,* 537–546, with permission from Elsevier LTD.)

have shown a quite normal response and awareness; one patient was able, using eye blinks, to write a book describing his thinking. In cases of locked-in syndrome, with the patient in a normal but almost completely inaccessible state of awareness, the PET measurements in Figure 7.2 show almost normal levels of brain energy consumption.[22] This additional correlation of high global energy and a high degree of awareness or consciousness supports high brain energy as a necessary attribute of such awareness. The high brain energy in the locked-in state shows that high brain energy is not sufficient for the state of consciousness, since my operational definition includes the ability to respond. In this practical definition only when patients were able to communicate by blinking did we become aware of their being in a state of consciousness. Additional cases where the ability to communicate is necessary for the state of consciousness to be acknowledged come from epileptics with high brain energy who do not satisfy our criteria for being in the state of consciousness.

These PET studies have reproducibly shown the reduction of global brain energy during the pathologies characterized by loss of consciousness. In reviewing these reproducible data, it is clear that proposals about the role of brain energy in the awake state of consciousness could be useful in interpreting and extending these clinical studies. It is at first somewhat surprising to read, in the extensive clinical literature accepting these results, that, although they seem to fulfill the research goal of finding a physical measurement that could replace subjective diagnosis of awareness, no effort has been reported about incorporating this parameter, which was the focus of their studies, into diagnosis. The hesitancy becomes understandable when we realize that to do so would be to acknowledge implicitly that a high level of brain energy consumption is a **necessary** property of the state of consciousness, a correlation that has only recently been proposed in the work I have been describing. The point that is missing in declaring that the loss of consciousness is caused by the reduced brain activity is that the high normal energy consumption is necessary to create the state of consciousness. If it were not necessary for the normal state of consciousness, then its reduced value during loss of consciousness could be an epiphenomenon, a fallout from some other cause of the loss. The hypothesis that high brain energy consumption is necessary for the person to be in a state of awareness can be tested in future patients, and if the data continue to support this diagnosis, it should carry weight in the hospital and the courtroom.

ROLE OF TOTAL ENERGY IN INTERPRETATIONS OF FMRI

fMRI experiments have been performed on patients with disorders of consciousness.[23] The fMRI maps of a large consort of patients diagnosed as in the vegetative or minimally conscious state have been evaluated to distinguish responses of the primary auditory cortex to auditory stimulation from any secondary, more subjective processing of the input information. All the patients showed activations of the primary auditory cortex. About half showed activated secondary regions, and the condition of these patients improved more after several months (as shown by the Coma Recovery Scale) than those patients without discernible secondary processes. The prognostic importance of the secondary fMRI responses highlights the importance of understanding the neuronal mechanisms responsible for the signal. Once again, the role of the baseline energy is relevant when planning treatment since, as described above, the magnitude of baseline energy consumption affects secondary fMRI signals. While the appearance of localization might argue for specific neuronal connections creating the secondary response, still, as we have seen, high global energy is necessary for this response, and its role must be explored before definite conclusions can be reached about the origin of the fMRI signal. A comprehensive basis for interpreting fMRI data and planning treatment of the disorders of consciousness will profit from the improved understanding of the role of local and global energies in the damaged brain.

Our pragmatic philosophy of neuroscience, in which brain measurements of energy consumption are correlated with observable behavior rather than with psychological terms, as applied to experiments on the correlation of sensory stimulation and perceptual awareness, offers an exciting future for distinguishing the roles of local and global contributions to normal and pathological brain functions.

NOTES

1. Craver, C. F. (2007). *Explaining the brain; mechanisms and the mosaic unity of neuroscience*. New York: Oxford University Press.
2. Bennett, M. R., & Hacker, P. M. S.(2003) *Philosophical foundations of neuroscience*. Malden, MA: Blackwell Publishing.
3. Ibid. (p. 244).
4. Zeman, A. (2002). *Consciousness: A user's guide* (pp. 16–18). New Haven, CT: Yale University Press.
5. Koch, C. (2004). *The quest for consciousness: A neurobiological approach* (pp. 17–19). Englewood, CO: Roberts & Co.
6. Op cit., Bennett & Hacker (p. 246).
7. Shulman, R. G., Hyder, F. H., & Rothman, D. L. (2009). Baseline brain energy supports the state of consciousness. *Proceedings of the National Academy of Sciences USA, 102*, 11096–11101.
8. Jarvilehto, T. (2009). The theory of the organism-environment system as basis of experimental work in psychology. *Ecological Psychology, 21*(2), 112–120.

9. Damasio, A. R. (1994). *Descartes' error: Emotion, reason, and the human brain* (p. xvii). New York: Putnam Publishing.

10. Hyder, F., Kida, I., Behar, K. L., Kennan, R. P., Maciejewski, P. K., & Rothman, D. L. (2001). Quantitative functional imaging of the brain: towards mapping neuronal activity by BOLD fMRI. *NMR Biomed., 14*(7–8), 413–431.

11. Smith, A. J., Blumenfeld, H., Behar, K. L., Rothman, D. L., Shulman, R. G., & Hyder, F. (2002). Cerebral energetics and spiking rates: The neurophysiological basis of fMRI. *Proceedings of the National Academy of Sciences USA, 99*(16), 10765–10770.

12. Maandag, N. J., Coman, D., Sanganahalli, B. G., Herman, P., Smith, A. J., Blumenfeld, H., Shulman, R. G., & Hyder, F. (2007). Energetics of neuronal signaling and fMRI activity. *Proceedings of the National Academy of Sciences USA, 104*(51), 20546–20551.

13. Franks, N. P. (2008). General anesthesia: from molecular targets to neuronal pathways of sleep and arousal. *Nature Review Neuroscience, 9*(5), 70–86.

14. Alkire, M. T., Haier, R. J., Barker, S. J., Shah, N. K., Wu, J. C., & Kao, Y. J. (1995). Cerebral metabolism during propofol anesthesia in humans studied with positron emission tomography. *Anesthesiology, 82*(2), 393–403; discussion 327A.

15. Alkire, M. T., & Miller, J. (2005). General anesthesia and the neural correlates of consciousness. *Prog. Brain Res., 150*, 229–244.

16. Kaisti, K. K., Langsjo, J. W., Aalto, S., Oikonen, V., Sipila, H., Teras, M., Hinkka, S., Metsahonkala, L., & Scheinin, H. (2003). Effects of sevoflurane, propofol, and adjunct nitrous oxide on regional cerebral blood flow, oxygen consumption, and blood volume in humans. *Anesthesiology, 99*(3), 603–613.

17. Alkire, M. T., Hudetz, A. G., & Tononi, G. (2008). Consciousness and anesthesia. *Science, 322*(5903), 876–880.

18. Alkire, M. T., Pomfrett, C. J., Haier, R. J., Gianzero, M. V., Chan, C. M., Jacobsen, B. P., & Fallon, J. H. (1999). Functional brain imaging during anesthesia in humans: effects of halothane on global and regional cerebral glucose metabolism. *Anesthesiology, 90*(3), 701–709.

19. Katoh, T., Bito, H., & Sato, S. (2000). Influence of age on hypnotic requirement, bispectral index, and 95% spectral edge frequency associated with sedation induced by sevoflurane. *Anesthesiology, 92*(1), 55–61.

20. Heinke, W., & Schwarzbauer, C. (2002). In vivo imaging of anaesthetic action in humans: approaches with positron emission tomography (PET) and functional magnetic resonance imaging (fMRI). *British Journal of Anaesthesiology, 89*(1), 112–122.

21. Laureys, S., & Schiff, N. D. (2012). Coma and consciousness: Paradigms (re)framed by neuroimaging. *Neuroimage, 61*, 476–491.

22. Laureys, S., Owen, A. M., Schiff, N. D. (2004). Brain function in coma, vegetative state, and related disorders. *Lancet Neurol. 3*, 537–546.

23. Coleman, M. R., Davis, M. H., Rodd, J. M., Robson, T., Ali, A., Owen, A. M., Pickard, J. D. (2009). Towards the routine use of brain imaging to aid the clinical diagnosis of disorders of consciousness. *Brain.132*, 2541–2552.

8

Incremental Brain Energies and
the Acts of Consciousness

I n neuroscience, the recurring problem of consciousness has been addressed as the need to establish the neural activities supporting consciousness in humans. The previous chapter referred to Bennett and Hacker's distinction between intransitive and transitive consciousness, and defined similar qualities as the state of consciousness and the acts of consciousness. However, the novel contribution made to this ongoing subject was not in renaming these phenomena but in showing that a high level of global, cortical energy (and its coupled neuronal activity) was necessary for the person to be in the state of consciousness. The assignment of high energy depended on noninvasive imaging results from PET and ^{13}CMRS. The state of consciousness was defined by behavior showing the human could respond to stimuli, following the anesthesiologist's criteria. High energy was a necessary brain property for that observable state but not sufficient, as shown by locked-in patients who could not respond by conventional means. Efforts to identify brain activities necessary for observable behavior will be continued in this chapter by exploring neuronal activities responsible for a person's performance of the acts of consciousness.

The acts of consciousness are the most evident manifestations of conscious recognition. Acts of consciousness similar to Bennett and Hacker's transitive consciousness are defined as "a matter of currently being conscious of something or conscious that something is thus-and-so."[1] In the act of consciousness the person knows something specific—that an event has been remembered or that an object has been moved from one place to another. The act of consciousness is a form of knowledge, and knowledge requires a prepared mind. To perform an act of consciousness, the person must be in the state of consciousness and additionally must have a relevant background or experience. By this definition, in the usual functional imaging experiment where a person compares and is conscious of the difference between two conditions, he performs an act of consciousness.

An act of consciousness is identified in an fMRI experiment by the person's perception, response, acknowledgement, denial, or agreement of the difference between two conditions as evidenced by his behavior. This definition of an act of consciousness allows us to vary the behavioral properties of these acts and to follow neuronal support of the person's acts by the fMRI signal. The response to a comparison depends upon the individual's history and experience as well as the experimental details. If the differences between the conditions are small, such as a sensory stimulus below the detectable level, or arcane, as in an unfamiliar language, they will not be noted and the incremental energies will be negligible since the conditions being compared will not be perceived as different. The fMRI signal is one measure of the differences in the neuronal energy that support the person's acknowledgment of the change between these conditions.

To the extent that differences, or their components, are recognized by the person and are repeatedly observable, as when normal individuals are exposed to sensory stimuli with specific properties of size, color, touch, or sound, then the brain response tends to be reproducible, as shown by fMRI signals. On repetition of a well-defined stimulus, the similar brain responses would, upon summation as is usually necessary in fMRI experiments, lead to a signal that is localized to the same region(s). On the other hand, to the extent that the difference recognized between the two conditions depended on poorly defined concepts, such as evaluating someone's intention, emotion, or other state of mind, which would vary with the experimental context, then the signal would generally not be repeatable; responses to subjective conditions have been shown to create not very reproducible activations of the parietal and prefrontal regions.[2] The experimental results illustrating the properties of the acts of consciousness in this chapter are of measured brain activities in the visual cortex during the person's changing awareness. We know what the person perceives by his behavior: he signals this awareness by raising one hand or by pushing a button. We identify brain activities needed for specific behaviors when the person has acknowledged perceiving one or another stimulus. However, and this is an important distinction between our definitions and those introduced by Cognitive Neuroscience, we do not try to define what the person is conscious of. Rees, Kreiman, and Koch,[2] reviewing this field, made a primary distinction between "the neural correlates of the **level** of consciousness (for example, awake, sleep, attentive or drowsy)" and "the neural correlates of specific phenomenological content (such as a green apple versus an orange)." The former definition corresponds to our state of consciousness and the latter to our acts of consciousness that are similar to Bennett and Hacker's. Although Rees and colleagues offer what seems like a similar breakdown of consciousness, it differs significantly from our state and acts of consciousness. Our acts of consciousness and states of consciousness are identified by a person's behavior, while Rees's are identified by descriptions or definitions of the objects, or concepts, whose brain correlates are sought. In their definition of a process similar to our acts of consciousness they have assumed that things like green apples (and consciousness) can be identified and that they are recognized by brain activities. As emphasized throughout the early chapters, we do not think it is possible to say that the brain does this, that, or the other thing. It is the person who distinguishes between green apples and oranges, and to say that the brain does so is to introduce a conceptualization that is meaningless. The pitfalls in the study of consciousness introduced by assigning to the brain the powers of recognizing concepts are evident when, if we followed the definitions of Rees and colleagues, we would find that to define neuronal correlates of consciousness we must first be able to define consciousness. This has led to the dead end of trying to identify qualia. Our behavioral definition avoided the psychological efforts that would be needed to define the mental processes assumed to underlie conceptualizations of consciousness. To introduce a concept of brain activity underlying behavior recognizing green apples (or consciousness) is like introducing a concept of memory when a person is observed to have remembered something. For a Pragmatist these concepts have no meaning and, as I have shown, experiments have not clarified them.

In the model of brain activity maintained in the earlier chapters, the imaging signal reflects the brain's role in serving the human behavior, like the muscle support of the groom's activity in lifting the bride across the threshold. We are able, in this view, to clearly recognize sensory stimuli because people are expert at distinguishing between horizontal and vertical lines or between a marriage ceremony and a football game because they understand how these activities are reproducibly and measurably different. The need for understanding in an act of consciousness can be tested by seeing how the fMRI signal is affected when a person is trained to become expert in a comparison about which he was formerly ignorant. When a person is taught to see a difference between two conditions, thereby distinguishing something that previously was a muddle, experimental results show that the brain response becomes a distinct, reproducible signal similar to the recognition of clear stimuli like horizontal or vertical lines. In these experiments, to be discussed below, signals in the visual cortex are changed when human subjects become experts in identifying visual stimuli that they previously could not distinguish and analogously change when a person's awareness switches from perceiving horizontal to vertical lines. However, before discussing fMRI signals revealing the role of awareness in neuroimages,

we must first recognize the present abilities and limitations of fMRI in identifying brain activities, and describe research directions that show promise of
improving our understanding of neuronal activity by fMRI.

NEURONAL BASIS OF FMRI ENERGETICS

The incremental signals measured by fMRI comparisons are the most novel
feature of neuroimaging experiments, and their ability to localize brain activities is mainly responsible for the broad interest generated by neuroimaging.
Calibrated fMRI can convert BOLD fMRI signals into incremental energies
that can provide a valuable experimental beginning for studying how neuronal
activities support a person's acts of consciousness. This approach is valuable
first to the extent we know the magnitudes and locations of BOLD signal's energies and second to the extent that these energies can be related quantitatively
to neuronal activities. Assuming, as I suggest, that the incremental energy can
lead us to the neural correlates of consciousness differs from the usual interpretations of the measured BOLD signal. Preliminary, selected studies of the
neuronal basis of fMRI signals in the rat were shown in Chapter 6, where histograms of firing rates in animals showed comparable increases in the relative
firing rates of a representative ensemble of neurons and the energies derivable
from calibrated fMRI signals. The equivalence of fMRI measurements of brain
energy and the rates of neuronal firing showed the value of energy for studying
brain functions. Since both incremental energies and baseline energies were
expressed in the same units, usually the metabolic rate of glucose oxidation,
it has been possible to combine their magnitudes, thereby obtaining the total
energies supporting acts of consciousness.[3]

The second limitation of present fMRI research has been the localizationist
view of mental activities that has been supported by the small number of activated voxels identified in fMRI experiments. This sparse measure of localized
activities contradicts the widely held view that mental activities emerge from
"complex, continuous whole-brain neuronal collaboration(s)" that is consistent
with the high global energy needed for brain function.[4] Gonzales-Castillo and
colleagues have addressed this discrepancy by an fMRI study utilizing massive
averaging to improve signal-to-noise and a model-free analysis that avoided
suggesting where activations were expected. In the absence of a model predicting localized activations, the averaging of a hundred repetitions of the same
subject's response to a simple visual stimulation and attention control task provided high signal-to-noise maps that showed activations distributed over 95%
of cortical gray matter. The authors suggested that a large number of responses
were found because the model-free assumptions did not limit the search to

regions expected from presumptions, while the many activations detected were allowed by the high signal-to-noise. Gonzales-Castillo and colleagues' innovative experiment shows that wide-ranging changes in neuronal activity mapped by fMRI (both increments and decrements) provide global brain support for the behavioral acts of consciousness.

For additional connections between the fMRI signal and the acts of consciousness, exemplifying the role played by the person's experiences, I turn to experiments showing how training a person to understand a comparison creates a modular brain response. These provide a connection between modular fMRI signals and the personal understanding or awareness needed for an act of consciousness.

FUSIFORM FACE AREA: DOWNSTREAM IN THE VISUAL CORTEX

The fusiform face area (FFA) of the human brain is a region in the anterior and middle fusiform gyri of the ventral visual cortex that was originally identified as responding to the sight of faces.[5] This regional brain response has been identified by fMRI, single-unit recording of neuronal responses, and by the consequences of lesions in humans and in nonhuman primates. At the beginning of 2011 there were more than 8,000 references to this intensely investigated area listed in PubMed. The fMRI difference signal identifying the FFA region is obtained by comparing the response to faces with that to different objects, including inverted faces.[6] The localized nature of the face response had led to questions about its function since it was hard to accept that these relatively large brain areas would be hardwired to exclusively detect faces. Two alternatives were proposed for the function of this region: either it specifically recognizes faces, or it responds to a variety of specialized processes of visual expertise and in addition to faces also recognizes other classes of objects such as animals, cars, or birds. The difference of opinion was soon settled by experiments with the harmonious answer that both parties are correct: it is now generally accepted that this region responds most strongly to the presentation of faces, but also can respond less strongly to animals, cars, tools, and a wide range of objects.[5,6]

fMRI images with higher spatial resolution divided the region into specialized subregions responding to cars, animals, or birds.[7] In accordance with the stronger response of the FFA to faces, there was a preponderance of regions with a preferential response to faces. Although details of the overlap of sub regions are still under study, the responses for all these objects, including faces, are subsumed by the larger FFA region, and the different sub regions are close to each other, if not actually superimposed.[8]

The fMRI results are supplemented by electrode measurements of populations of neurons and of single neurons. Studies of the fine structure of the face recognition region have shown that the topography of the neural code for faces and objects exists at multiple spatial scales.[9] The regions ranged from the relatively coarse scale of an fMRI voxel, first reported by Puce and colleagues,[10] that averaged responses from thousands of neurons, down to a finer scale selective for a population of neurons, and finally, at the finest scale (where electrode measurements of single neurons replaced fMRI signals), to a level where individual neurons are tuned to different preferred categories.[11] At all these levels the activations are spread across populations, of voxels or neurons, similar in their diffuse spatial response and in their broad selectivity to stimuli. From the fMRI voxel down to the single neuron, the brain responses are broadly localized and broadly tuned.

EXPERTISE

Although this region's localized response to objects is not completely understood at the neuronal level, research reports have agreed that expertise is a strong factor leading to specialization of the FFA. The role of expertise was shown in an innovative early experiment[12] that started by localizing the FFA region in the standard way by the large difference signal between the fMRI signal from a face and an inverted face. In a cohort of untrained human subjects, there was only a small difference signal obtained when the response from an inverted Greeble, a class of novel head-like objects, was subtracted from the response of a right-side-up Greeble. However, after the same human subjects were trained to identify Greebles, the difference signal between right-side-up and inverted Greebles became almost as large as for human faces. The expertise for novel objects, like Greebles, developed by training created responses in the right medial FFA that were almost as large as the normal response to faces at the customary fMRI spatial resolution.

These results show that human experiences, such as our continual exposure to faces, can act as top-down forces on the sensory selectivity. This strong interaction between the individual's experience and his sensory perception shows it cannot be assumed that regional responses are built-in or intrinsic. My ability to distinguish Chevrolets from BMWs is supported by a sparse population of neurons and voxels and has required my expertise in identifying cars that has been developed in a social context and by other personal experiences. The ability to distinguish automobiles is not a universal human property but is very useful for a particular population. The strengthened neuronal responses to an individual's interests, evidenced by expertise, show how the individual trains the brain, not vice versa. The difference between the modularity of the sensory response and the rather delocalized response to higher-order concepts reflects the person's more precise understanding of the former. They are inconsistent with the claims made by cognitive psychologists that "The brain made me do it."[13] Rather, they show that brain activity not only influences behavior by conveying stimuli but also responds to it by its plasticity.

REPRODUCIBLE RESPONSES OF SENSORY STIMULI

The usual observation in fMRI studies that sensory responses are distinct has, in our previous discussion, paid little attention to the evidence that sensory responses are strongly influenced by the individual's history of interactions with his environment, as shown in the Greebles experiment. However, it had early been shown by Hubel and Weisel[14] that sensory deprivation and enhancement, particularly during early formative years, created, modified, or disrupted specific sensory inputs. (For excellent reviews of brain plasticity created by sensory experiences, see Note 15.) Experiments on animals that were reared in the dark, or with one eye blocked, showed extensive cellular, structural, and functional changes of the visual pathway. In the retina and the lateral geniculate and immediate cortical areas, the cellular densities, sizes, and connections were all drastically altered by deprivation of light. In animals deprived of the view of right-moving lines, ~90% of the neurons, which in the control animal are equally likely to respond to right or left, responded only to the left-moving lines. Similarly reproducible responses of the normally raised animal to vertical or horizontal lines, to color, and to upside-down or right-side-up views are distorted in the adults who were sensory-deprived as youngsters. The detailed breakdown of the visual input is dependent upon experience, particularly during early exposures.[15] Similar, although less severe, changes were reported for sensory deprivation during later developmental times. The interdependent effects of sensory deprivation, enrichment, and experience on brain structure and function led Bruce Wexler, an advocate of plasticity, to assert that "The relationship between the individual and the environment is so extensive that it almost overstates the distinction between the two to speak of a relationship at all."[16] In summary, the difference between the distinctiveness of the sensory response and the rather delocalized response to higher-order concepts is a consequence of the person's more definite understanding of the former. In the present example, learning to distinguish Greebles has been identified by the subject's behavior, and the brain support of recognizing an object has been manifested by the FFA response. The distinctiveness of a response presumably can be helped by neuroanatomy, but, as shown by rewired animal brains, training and experience can overcome the need for a specific neural anatomy.[15]

BINOCULAR RIVALRY

The Greebles results show that consistent fMRI responses in the FFA are observed when a person learns to recognize certain objects, demonstrating that activities in the visual cortex are coupled to the person's demonstrable understanding. The response to vision starts with retinal input to region V1 of the visual cortex in the back of the brain, followed by brain responses in regions beyond V1 in the downstream extrastriate visual cortex (which covers more than one quarter of the human cortex and includes the FFA region) to components of the visual stimuli like color or motion. To supplement the specific response of FFA we now turn to experiments that have shown correlations of behavioral awareness with activities throughout the visual cortex. These experiments, led by studies of binocular rivalry, are beginning to answer the question as to what extent bottom-up measurements of reliable sensory responses can reveal brain processes supporting human behavior.

Awareness of an object may be defined behaviorally by the ability of a subject to report its presence. Based on imaging and other studies, the ability to be aware involves brain regions that do not directly receive sensory input, such as the frontal lobes. An act of consciousness by definition requires that the subjects are aware of the act they are performing. The study of the impact of conscious awareness on primary sensory regions has been pioneered by the binocular rivalry experiments of Nikos Logothetis and David Leopold, who traced the changing neuronal activations as the monkey's awareness of a signal switched from one eye to the other.[17,18] When monkeys were presented simultaneously with a different image to each eye, their awareness, as reported by the subjects and indicated by their behavior, switched back and forth between the two images. When steadily presented with horizontal stripes to one eye and vertical stripes to the other, their awareness switched between horizontal and vertical lines, in accord with reported awareness, rather than consisting of the crosshatched pattern that would be expected from a superimposition of the two inputs.

Leopold and Logothetis measured the neuronal firing throughout the brain as the monkeys signaled their awareness of either horizontal or vertical lines by pulling levers. Increases in the firing rates of specific neurons throughout the brain coincided with the animal's awareness of each input. They reported that although a large fraction of the neurons in the visual cortex fired independently of the state of awareness, still "the activity of nearly all visually responsive neurons in areas IT and STS closely matched the animal's perceptive state." And they proposed that "reorganizations of activity throughout the visual cortex, concurrent with perceptual reversals, are initiated by higher, largely non-sensory brain centers."[17]

The significance of the rivalry studies has led many investigators to study the phenomenon using a variety of methods. fMRI results showed a similar, but not identical, correspondence in humans with the monkey's correlations of neuronal activities with perception.[19,20] Correlations of activities with awareness were found in all regions of the visual cortex by fMRI, including V1 when the rival signals were of strongly differing contrast.[20] fMRI studies differ qualitatively from the monkey multi-unit recordings that showed weaker correlations with awareness in the V1 and V2 regions by showing significant correlations of the early V1 and V2 areas with awareness, but they qualitatively agree with the firing results, under the initial conditions, by showing larger fractions of correlated neurons as one moves down the visual pathway.

BOLD FMRI ENERGY AND NEURONAL FIRING

The differences between neurophysiological measurements of neuronal firing rates and the BOLD fMRI signals in the V1 and V2 regions has led to an intense search for the neuronal meaning of BOLD fMRI signals. In resolving this inconsistency in the higher visual cortex Logothetis has, on the basis of a slightly better statistical fit to the data,[21] assigned the physical origin of the fMRI signal to the local field potentials (LFPs), denying that fMRI signals are a measure of firing rates. The search to unify all these valid results has been complicated by the diverse nature of the parameters measured by different techniques. The multi-unit recordings measure the neuronal firing rates, the fMRI measure a combination of CBF, $CMRO_2$, and cerebral blood volume, while the LFPs measure an unspecifiable result of many neuronal activities. Our suggestion that energy can be a unifying parameter for different measurements has been directed toward resolving these comparisons. Results in our laboratory have been deriving the consumption of energy from fMRI, MRS, and PET experiments and relating it to the work of neurotransmission. The ^{13}CMRS experiments showed that the energy of oxidizing glucose was dedicated to the work of processes associated with synaptic activity as judged by glutamate neurotransmitter release. In a recent review this correlation between the measured glucose oxidation and the energy dedicated to neuronal activity, originally based on rat data, has been extended to human brain results.[22]

Correlations between the energy dedicated to glutamate neurotransmitter release and the rate of neuronal firing in the rat have been shown in Chapter 6.

To the extent that these correlations between energy consumption and neuronal firing rates can be made quantitative, the fMRI results, when calibrated to obtain energy, can be directly converted to neuronal firing rates. In this way the separate advantages of fMRI and multi-unit recordings of firing rates can be combined into a comprehensive understanding of the brain responses to the acts of consciousness.

However, there are experimental results that hinder the direct conversion of energy consumption to the work of neuronal firing. The first, which has been answered by the ^{13}CMRS experiments in rats, and brought to human applications recently, is the question as to how much of the energy of the synaptic activity revealed by glutamate neurotransmissions cycling is devoted to firing. That has been shown to be about 80% in the resting rat and somewhat less but still a strong majority in the human. The second objection is more persistent: namely, how much of the energy accompanying the synaptic activity, as measured by glutamate cycling, is devoted to firing because the use of that energy for inhibitory processes has been shown, in certain examples, not to be negligible.[23-25] Both the excitatory firings of glutamatergic synapses and the inhibitory synaptic processes mediated by gamma-amino-butyric acid (GABA) contribute to the glutamate release and cycling measured in ^{13}CMRS, requiring separate measurements before energy can be converted to firing rates.

The inhibitory GABA processes can be separated from the excitatory glutamatergic activities in other ^{13}CMRS experiments by using a differently labeled glucose and have been shown[26] in the somatosensory regions of the rat cortex to consume ~20% of the total energy. Measurements of the fractional contributions of inhibitory processes are not limited to the somatosensory cortex and could evaluate the inhibitor energy consumption throughout the brain. These additional experiments can provide a quantitative relationship between energy and neuronal firing wherever needed. On the other hand, it may be said that the importance of neuronal firing versus synaptic energy consumption is model-dependent, based on the assumption that firing will lead to an understanding of brain function. The slight decoupling between energy consumption and firing (that can be evaluated by these measurements of GABA activity) raises the question as to whether energy consumption, quantitatively measuring the sum of excitatory and inhibitory synaptic activity, is perhaps a more valuable parameter of brain function than is firing. Nonetheless, to the extent that present theories of brain function depend on neurons communicating by excitatory firings, the relationship between neuronal energy consumption and the excitatory firing can be quantitated by extending the GABA ^{13}CMRS to cortical areas of interest. The energies from calibrated fMRI and ^{13}CMRS that can be assigned to firing (after correcting for contributions from GABA) can provide brain activities responding to the acts of consciousness with a firm thermodynamic base.

BRAIN WORK SUPPORTS THE PERSON

Elegant experiments frame a neuronal model between activations in the prefrontal-parietal region by the subjective act of consciousness and signals in the extra striate visual cortex that delineate a mechanism by which brain activity responds to and supports the person's behavior. In conformity with the findings of Logothetis and Leopold,[18] Geraint Rees, Gabriel Kreiman, and Christof Koch[2] traced the neuronal pathway of acts of consciousness throughout the human brain from visual stimulation. In a subsequent summary of several reports, Koch and Rees[27] showed that in a number of experiments the broad responses in parietal and prefrontal regions correlated with a subject's awareness and, in support of an earlier suggestion by Crick and Koch,[28] showed that this region plays a prominent role in the pathways of consciousness. The direction of information flow from awareness was inferred from the time courses of fMRI activations, suggesting that the parietal-prefrontal response preceded the changes that awareness introduced into the visual cortex.[29]

This direction of flow, from the person's behavior to brain activity, was shown directly by the expertise experiments where training improved the person's recognition of Greebles. In concordance with the binocular rivalry experiments, fMRI has shown that as human awareness switches to responding to a face from a vase in an ambivalent face/vase picture, the modular fMRI activations become stronger in the FFA region.[30] As the physical meaningfulness of these neurophysiological experiments is clarified by experimentation, we can expect to see fMRI fulfill its potential for more fully describing brain activities necessary for the behavioral acts of consciousness.

These reliable neuronal and behavioral experiments justify the hopes in Chapter 6 (and the explicit goals of neurophysiology) that bottom-up studies can make progress in relating neuronal energies and activities to observable behavior. Mental processes during identifiable behavior have been observed without introducing nonphysical assumptions. By regarding energy as a parameter and combining the incremental energies with the total or baseline brain energy, the fMRI BOLD signals can be extended to provide a quantitative comparison of the energy and neuronal firing during the two conditions of an fMRI experiment.

TOWARD AN EMPIRICAL PSYCHOLOGY

A goal of this book was to describe how neuronal processes could reliably be identified with behavior, thereby avoiding the uncertainties introduced by psychological generalizations presumed to underlie that behavior. The binocular rivalry experiment is an elegant example of the reliability that can be found for both experimental parameters. In contemplating how these results may be correlated with other acts of consciousness, I propose that a pragmatic philosophy is needed, where a description of observable behavior would be treated as a hypothesis whose generality is to be tested. The imaging results can help test the validity of an empirical psychology. Psychology relates individual, personal acts to general principles, directly facing the interplay of subjective and objective phenomenon. Cognitive psychology was a positivistic effort to address these goals, and in its place I suggest that a more flexible psychology where both behavior and the general principles to which it is attributed should be more flexible, more susceptible to pragmatic modification. I cannot endorse a particular psychology: that would be beyond the scope of this review.

However, the neuronal data by which such psychological concepts are to be judged is within our scope, and the advantages that our interpretation of neuronal experiments have over some accepted views merit summation. We have been proposing that neuroimaging data, including fMRI, can yield values of energy consumption that can be converted to neuronal firing, the basis of awareness in electrode experiments. Using energy to relate fMRI to awareness differs from popular interpretations of experimental results. Sterzer, Kleinschmidt, and Rees, in a review of the neural bases of multistable perception, follow reports[31] that fMRI signals do not give firing but give values of LFP. They further suggest that LFP, not neuronal firing, is a measure of awareness. In place of these phenomenological correlations of LFP, I have described how quantitative relations between firing rates, energy, and the influence of top-down awareness on sensory neuronal responses can provide a reliable physical basis for evaluating psychological processes.

BRAIN SUPPORT OF ADAPTATION

The experimental data reviewed above are consistent with my criticisms of several popular theories of brain function. It's not as the computer scientists suggest that the brain's function is to process information; nor as the cognitive psychologists suggest does it represent specific behavior by general concepts; nor as some economists suggest is it capable of making a rational choice; nor as linguists posit does it have intrinsic language capabilities. Rather, the data show that brain activity supports the person's interests, responding reproducibly to a person's understanding in his act of consciousness. The brain helps the person to perform many functions. In this sense the brain is similar to many properties needed for survival. Like our visual acuity, our upright posture, or our slow development into adulthood, it creates a condition that helps the individual to survive. The brain, like the opposed thumb, enables the person to do many things: to pick up pennies, to hold on when climbing, and to throw a spear accurately.

In understanding how the total and incremental brain energies support the person's behavior and experience, we begin to understand the mechanisms by which brain function serves adaptation. In supporting human responses to the world, brain function can be understood as an adaptation that "evolved because it improved survival and reproductive performance."[32] The brain is adaptive and has helped the human species to survive not because it was intended to do that—but because it did, we find it to have survived.

Evolution is such a comprehensive explanation of biological phenomena that it could be asked of this overall view of brain function why isn't it just an assumption at the beginning of the book—after all, every human property that we can observe has survived and therefore is an aspect of human adaptation, so the brain should not be an exception. The answer to this possible criticism is that we have shown **how** brain energy consumption does the work of neuronal firing that has been used by the individual to fulfill the needs of consciousness. We have presented the mechanisms by which energy from the oxidation of glucose has been used in two different forms to support two different observable components of conscious behavior. The global total energy provides necessary support for the person to be in the state of consciousness, an observable state identified by his ability to respond to stimuli. Analogously, the incremental energies observed in fMRI and PET experiments have identified brain activities that help a person respond to the environment by building on previous experiences. fMRI provides a start for measuring brain locations of the additional energy spent in recognizing faces or horizontal lines and other brain activities that prepare the person for recurrent experiences. The neuronal activation in response to sensory inputs is not, as cognitive psychologists among others have suggested, an intrinsic brain property, but a brain function that supports the individual's variegated efforts to understand the world.

The importance of having arrived at these conclusions by delineating the mechanisms of energy support for the human ability to survive is revealed by a contrasting statement made in the early pages of this book. Repeating a commonly accepted position since Claude Bernard first enunciated it, I agreed that "Physical scientists can find necessary explanations of how things happen at the chemical or physical level, but they cannot justify these explanations by appealing to a higher authority because there is no higher authority than physical and chemical explanations."[33] Reliability is sacrificed if we build on other than physical assumptions—such as those arising in psychology or linguistics. The present text criticized many functional imaging experiments because they are built on assumptions that do not have the validity of physical science. However, even though adaptation as a condition for evolutionary survival has a lot of traction—more generally believed than other nonphysical claims—still a bland assertion that the brain, like everything human, serves adaptation does not convey the meaningfulness offered by our argument that brain work is supported by energy consumption. The important claim made in these pages is that physical scientific results describe mechanisms by which the brain helps the person to live his life, and if we seek a larger narrative into which those individual impulses can be located, it would be in the successful drive to use one's tools, including the brain, to improve survivability and procreation.

NOTES

1. Bennett, M. R., & Hacker, P. M. S. (2003). *Philosophical foundations of neuroscience* (p. 248). Malden, MA: Blackwell Publishing. If one could measure the firing rates and other properties of all the excitatory and inhibitory neurons during both conditions in an fMRI experiment, they would describe neuronal activities necessary for the person to be aware of the differences between the two conditions. In this event, the difference between the total neuronal activities in the two conditions would be an unnecessary concept because it would have been identified by the total energies describing the state of consciousness. However, this would relinquish the opportunity to begin studies with the incremental activities available from fMRI, as discussed below, and the total activities measured by PET and MRS, as described in the last chapter.
2. Rees, G., Kreiman, G., & Koch, C. (2002). Neural correlates of consciousness in humans. *Nature Reviews Neuroscience, 3*, 261–270.
3. Shulman, R. G., & Rothman, D. L. (1998). Interpreting functional imaging studies in terms of neurotransmitter cycling. *Proceedings of the National Academy of Sciences USA, 95*, 11993–11998.
4. Gonzalez-Castillo, J., Saad, Z. S., Handwerker, D. A., Inati, S. J., Brenowitz, N., & Bandettini, P. A. (2012). Whole-brain, time-locked activation with simple tasks revealed using massive averaging and model-free analysis. Interpreting functional imaging studies in terms of neurotransmitter cycling. *Proceedings of the National Academy of Sciences USA, 109*(14), 5487–5492.
5. For a review see Peissig, J. J., & Tarr, M. T. (2007). Visual object recognition: Do we know more now than we did 20 years ago? *Annual Rev. Psychol., 58*, 75–96.
6. Downing, P. E., Chan, A. W. Y., Peelen, M. V., Dodds, C. M., & Kanwisher, N. (2006). Domain specificity in visual cortex. *Cerebral Cortex, 16*, 1453–1461.
7. Gauthier, I., Skudlarski, P., Gore, J. C., & Anderson, A. W. (2000). Expertise for cars and birds recruits brain areas involved in face recognition. *Nature Neuroscience, 3*, 191–197.
8. Grill-Spector, K., Sayres, R., & Ress, D. (2006). High-resolution imaging reveals highly selective non-face clusters in the fusiform face area. *Nature Neuroscience, 9*, 1177–1185. (Erratum in: *Nature Neuroscience* (2007), *10*(1), 133.)

9. Haxby, J. V. (2006). Fine structure in representations of faces and objects. *Nature Neuroscience, 9,* 1084–1086.
10. Puce, A., Allison, T., Gore, J. C., & McCarthy, G. (1995). Face-sensitive regions in extra-striate cortex studied by functional fMRI. *J. Neurophysiol., 74,* 1192–1190.
11. Logothetis, N. K., & Pauls, J. (1995). Psychophysical and physiological evidence for reviewer centered object recognition in the primate. *Cerebral Cortex, 5,* 270–288.
12. Gauthier, I., Tarr, M. J., Anderson, A. W., Skudlarski, P., & Gore, J. C. (1999). Activation of the middle fusiform 'face area' increases with expertise in recognizing novel objects. *Nature Neuroscience, 2,* 568–573.
13. Gazzaniga, M. (2005). My brain made me do it. In M. Gazzaniga (Ed.), *The ethical brain* (pp. 87–105). New York: Dana Press.
14. Hubel, D. H. (1988). *Eye, brain and vision.* New York: Scientific American Library.
15. Begley, S. (2008). *Train your mind, change your brain* (p. 48). New York: Ballantine Books.
16. Wexler, B. E. (2006). *Brain and culture: Neurobiology, ideology and social change.* Cambridge, MA: A Bradford Book, The MIT Press.
17. Leopold, D., & Logothetis, N. K. (1999). Multistable phenomena: changing views in perception. *Trends in Cognitive Science, 3,* 254–264.
18. Leopold, D. A., & Logothetis, N. K. (1996). Activity changes in early visual cortex reflect monkeys percepts during binocular rivalry. *Nature, 379,* 549–553.
19. Lumer, E. D., Friston, K. J., & Rees, G. (1998). Neural correlates of perceptual rivalry in the human brain. *Science, 280,* 1980–1984.
20. Polonsky, A., Blake, R., Braun, J., & Heeger, D. J. (2000). Neuronal activity in human primary visual cortex correlates with perception during binocular rivalry. *Nature Neuroscience, 3,* 1153–1159.
21. Magri, C., Schridde, U., Murayama, Y., Panzeri, S., & Logothetis, N. K. (2012). The amplitude and timing of the BOLD signal reflects the relationship between local field potential power at different frequencies. *J. Neurosci., 32,* 1395–1407.
22. Hyder, F., Rothman D. L., & Bennett, M.(2013) *Proceedings of the National Academy of Sciences USA,* accepted (private communication)..
23 Logothetis, N. K.,& Pfeuffer, J. (2004). On the nature of the BOLD fMRI contrast mechanism. *Magnetic Resonance Imaging, 22,* 1517–1531.
24. Heeger, D. J., & Ress, D. (2002). What does fMRI tell us about neuronal activity? *Nature Reviews Neuroscience, 3,* 1142–1151.
25 Tong, F., Meng, M., & Blake, R. (2006). Neural bases of binocular rivalry. *Trends in Cognitive Science, 10,* 502–511.
26. Patel, A. B., de Graaf, R. A., Mason, G. F., Rothman, D. L., Shulman, R. G., and Behar, K. L. (2005). The contribution of GABA to glutamate/glutamine cycling and energy metabolism in the rat cortex *in vivo. Proceedings of the National Academy of Sciences USA, 102,* 5588–5593
27. Koch, C., & Rees, G. (2007). Neural correlates of the contents of visual awareness in humans. *Phil. Trans. R. Soc. Lond. B Biol. Sci., 362*(1481), 877–886.
28. Crick, F., & Koch, C. (1998). Consciousness and neuroscience. *Cerebral Cortex, 8,* 97–107.
29. Sterzer, P., & Kleinschmidt, A. (2007). A neural basis for inference in perceptual ambiguity. *Proceedings of the National Academy of Sciences USA, 104,* 323–328.

30. Hasson, U., Hendler, T., Ben Bashat, D., & Malach, R. (2001). Vase or face? A neural correlate of shape-selective grouping processes in the human brain. *J. Cogn. Neurosci., 13,* 744–753.

31. Sterzer, P., Kleinschmidt, A., & Rees, G. (2009). The neural bases of multistable perception. *Trends in Cognitive Science, 13,* 310–318.

32. Stearns, S. C., & Hoekstra, R. F. (2000). *Evolution: an introduction* (p. 13). New York: Oxford University Press.

33. Bernard, C. (1957). *An introduction to the study of experimental medicine* (Transl. H. C. Greene, p. 66). New York: Dover Publications.

Epilogue

A Life in Humanities and Science

I once overheard one undergraduate consoling another: "Be philosophical," he said, "Don't think about it." Although this usage extended Webster's definition of remaining "rationally or sensibly calm under trying circumstances," it remains an apt description of many scientists' approach to the philosophical topics that undergird their daily work. Few scientists would deny that philosophy influences science, and most would confidently assert that a useful philosophy for science is now firmly in place, so there is no need to think about revising it or, in fact, even to think about it. Physicists, chemists, and the more physically oriented biologists follow a philosophy that values empirical tests of hypotheses so that now, after centuries of testing, there is rather broad acceptance about the nuts and bolts of everyday scientific practice. Traditional philosophy of science, based upon the great scientist-philosophers (Descartes, Galileo, Newton, von Helmholtz, and Bernard), has guided physical scientists through metaphysical issues by clarifying the role of experimentation and hypothesis.

However, when physical scientists turn to experimental studies of brain function, they encounter areas of investigation that require tools that reach beyond their usual epistemological boundaries. This different range of investigation is worth pausing on for just a moment. Philosophy that serves as the basis for scientific investigation (centuries in the making) goes relatively unquestioned by those who are practicing science. When those scientists turn from measuring the energy of particles or the structure of an oligonucleotide to asking, "How do we remember something?" or "What makes us cry?" they are leaving the epistemological framework that they use to analyze physical matter.

They then move to new fields where they are brought face to face with metaphysical issues such as mind, consciousness, and memory. They will find there (as they would if they spoke about such issues with friends or family, let alone with philosophers or psychologists) conflicting claims about how these concepts describe the world. It is the premise of this book that reliance on a traditional metaphysical philosophy of mind, in general, proves to be misleading for the practice of neuroscience. Traditional philosophies of mind are generally not inductions from empirical studies of the physical world but are responses to matters that philosophers have been defining and redefining since Descartes. Since these philosophical propositions have been incorporated into everyday life, scientists who set out to find objective descriptions of brain activities and function are, as members of our culture, trapped in an existing web of subjective, philosophical opinions. The goal of this book is to provide one form of guidance for scientists hoping to disentangle the objective goals of scientific study from the complex, fascinating, and generally unscientific understandings of the human condition that are accepted by all of us living within a given culture.

As I wrote this book, I would occasionally find myself explaining—to friends or to myself—how I, as a lifelong physical scientist, was making an argument that some would read as belittling the power of our science. I could tell that some were hearing—and fearing—that I'd turned "relativist"—that my time living in the academy had seduced me into thinking that science's claims were uncertain, slippery, the product of society's "power structures." I could feel that some of my scientist friends were dumbfounded—confused as to why I was anything but gleeful by the amount of progress that our science had made and was making. How did I get to this point of questioning, from within, a field of research that I have worked my whole life to help build? My story is one of a biophysicist, whose noninvasive magnetic resonance experiments on metabolism in yeast and skeletal muscle led me into brain studies and questions about the mind. I was, like so many others, intrigued at first because of the obvious allure of being able to apply scientific research to such fascinating questions as mind and memory. When these experiments started giving unreliable results, I could have turned away from the neuroimaging experiments of cognitive terms and shrugged it off as a bad path. But the high claims of cognitive psychology triggered some of my nonprofessional feelings, my personal sense of what makes human life as rich as it is; I found it difficult to accept the implications of cognitive psychology that the nuanced panoply of human feelings involved in such personal activities as remembering, intending, planning, and thinking all could be reduced to an automatic computer-like responses that could be read by the brain as algorithms. My determination to clarify the psychology behind the contradictory imaging results was only partly built on a respect for clean-cut scientific findings, which I had lived for as a dedicated scientist. It also reflected a lifetime of personal commitments to the importance of complex humanistic undertakings—our capacity to make and appreciate art or literature or to have and manage complex personal thoughts—as the basis of a meaningful life. I believe that these values were what led me to question what I was seeing, and the roots of this worldview—a view that prevented me from mindlessly

following the drumbeat of the current scientific milieu without questioning—
started in my early schooldays.

FORMATIVE YEARS—FAR ROCKAWAY AND
COLUMBIA COLLEGE

To the extent that any part of a story is memorable and separable, there was a
conspicuous early step in my path to science. I was in the school bus going to
Far Rockaway High School and two boys behind me were vivaciously criticizing poetry, politics, and movies and gossiping about actors. I turned around and
said something like, "You guys know an awful lot. How do you know all this?"
One of them was Howard Moss, who said, "Oh, we're intellectuals." I decided
right then and there at age 13 that I wanted to be "an intellectual." As the twig
is bent, that is what I have been for the many years since. Howard went on to
be an honored poet and nurtured poetry for many years as poetry editor of *The
New Yorker*.

Soon afterwards I went to Columbia College with a Pulitzer Prize scholarship, a legacy from a nineteenth-century publisher dedicated to exposing New
York City public school boys to the inner realms of Western culture available at
Columbia. A friend of mine had received that same scholarship a year earlier
and had lent me the books that were read in Columbia's humanities course for
freshman. I had time before enrolling, so I read that curriculum from Homer
onward and immediately knew I was hooked. In the first year of the humanities
class my expectations were raised even further by the good fortune of having
Lionel Trilling as teacher. Reading and discussing under his guidance was a
miraculous education as he courteously responded to students' passionate but
rudimentary questions on the readings by gently locating their unformed ideas
in the great traditions of St. Augustine or Kant that the course itself was exploring. In response to his teaching we felt reassured of having the right to join that
tradition as long as we were curious, and as long as we cared about what we
were doing.

But then toward the midterm, a problem developed when a new method
was announced for the midterm exam. Questions were to be given a week
in advance, and students would have to prepare answers to all the questions
because some would be selected for the midterm exam. I stood up and criticized this proposal, pointing out how intolerable it was that instead of rewarding creativity or the ability to respond to a challenge, this plan was rewarding
work, real drudgery, and I didn't want to be judged on that basis. I was heard
out, but the exam went on as planned with several questions, one of which
asked what Montaigne and Shakespeare thought about education. I responded

in one short sentence that "they both were for it." I then quoted something from Montaigne, and said in one more sentence that the plays we had read (*Henry IV, Parts 1 and 2*) were all about the education of Prince Hal. So I left Lionel with the question of what grade I was going to get. I got a B⁺, which in those days was not an F under another name; it was a real grade. Nonetheless (or maybe because of this difference), we soon became very friendly. We played tennis and he talked to me about the perfect fit offered by Brooks Bothers shirts. For the 16-year-old it was a heady entrance into the dazzling world that Columbia guarded.

In refusing to accept the changed midterm examination I was, for an undergraduate, demanding an unusual degree of autonomy. Lionel appreciated the generative force in literature of this tension. In his great essay "Freud: Within and Beyond Culture,"[1] he wrote: "The function of literature, through all its mutations, has been to make us aware of the particularity of selves, and the high authority of the self in its quarrel with its society and its culture. Literature is in that sense subversive." The opposing pulls of the world and the individual were not to be avoided or judged but rather to be appreciated as the deepest commitments to being human. The similar appreciation of opposites brought him to avoid and condemn any commitment to either end of a dyad, a balanced position that formed his literary and political expressions, and was not a style but a vision of the human condition. In later life, recognizing Lionel's continual and explicit defense of the individual from the claims of a culture that he admired and appreciated, I began to understand how I had shared, naïvely and unknowingly, Lionel's concerns about the demands made upon the individual's essential uniqueness by the culture around him. On the other hand, it was in the image of that culture, of the great books we read and the great discussions of them, that I was recreating myself. Perhaps it was my simultaneous resistance to the demands of the midterm exam contrasted with my wholehearted acceptance of the course contents that played a role in bringing him to befriend me as a young student.

Lionel Trilling did not advise a difficult path of subversion for the young science major but suggested that a career path as a historian of science would harmonize with his interests. However I chose the path of physics and chemistry, because they offered more obdurate opportunities for self-expression than the study of its history, which, at the time, seemed more like a passive retelling of progress. This idealistic view of science had been nurtured by the broader culture of my early years. In movies Paul Muni portrayed Pasteur's successes and Edward G. Robinson finally found Dr. Ehrlich's magic bullet on his 606th try, while in Bell's "Men of Mathematics" young doomed mathematicians embodied the romantic ideal that poetry found in Keats and Shelley. Nor was it an exaggeration to appreciate the heroic nature of modern physical science symbolized by Copernicus, Galileo, and Newton, who had challenged religious dogmatism and created the modern world with its hopes of enlightened reason. I had found a culture that I admired and embraced, and that also gave me the right venue for expressing and defining myself.

THE WHITNEY HUMANITIES CENTER

After 30 years of conducting experimental science in the laboratory, I reentered a broad culture of the humanities when I joined the Yale faculty in 1979. Once again, as during my early years at Columbia, I was fortunate at Yale to encounter and eventually to participate in a vibrant center of humanist activity. At Yale the humanities departments were living under the fundamental questioning of their viability that had been fomented, locally, by Paul De Man, who had been the leader of the American version of the deconstructionist movement imported from France. Recognizing the power but also the frustrations and nihilistic possibilities of the extremes of the skeptical approach, Bart Giamatti and Peter Brooks formed at Yale the Whitney Humanities Center, which soon housed a brilliant faculty fellowship that I was privileged to join. Each week, at the lunch meetings, a paper was presented at the Humanities Center that would generate far-ranging discussions. Very differently from an everyday conversation and from a scientific meeting, words were examined in careful tones like scientific specimens. A continual examination prevailed of the values and directions of literature and its criticism in the aftermath of deconstructionism. In some ways, this collective weighing of the allowable limits of literature and its criticism continued the self-examination that Trilling had inspired in me. The Whitney Humanities Center relit an interest that 30 years in suburban New Jersey had not fully quenched. I soon understood, in the words that Peter Brooks used, "the seriousness of literature."

The Whitney Humanities Center reflected the intellectual and political forces of its place and time. Before its formation in 1982 the Yale literature department was dominated by deconstructionism, which because of its free-floating range of activities defies a rigorous definition. At the core of its wide reach, deconstructionism questioned the existing definitions and practices of literature and literary criticism. In this rebellious position, traditional assumptions about the meaning of a text or a word or a thought were open to question, and of course the questioning itself had very few bounds. It held what seemed like extreme positions—such as that the author had no right to describe the text; that was up to the reader—and it began to seem that there was nothing in books, words, and the thoughts they invoked that could escape questioning. In its skeptical criticism of literary values and their implicit philosophical positions, deconstructionism and its many offshoots were manifestations of the uprisings against traditional authorities on the campuses and in the political world of its time. The uniqueness of these literary movements—deconstruction, semiotics, structuralism, and their derivatives—was their grounding in the discipline of literature. At times practitioners struck out boldly, sometimes recklessly, into other fields—movies, gender studies, and sexuality—but their apparent diffuseness was gathered in by their literary origins. At the core of this apparently free-ranging attitude was a self-criticism— students of literature were questioning the tenets of their field. I don't know how it happened, and I have not seen any history of the Whitney Humanities Center that could have traced this development, but somehow the freedom and value offered by self-criticism, not of the individual but of his discipline, became the guiding spirit of the Whitney Humanities Center. But, in contrast to the revolutionary spirit of the earlier deconstructionists, the fellows at the Humanities Center were rather conservatively committed to their disciplines. They were not trying to discard or overturn their fields; rather, by using the skeptical insights of the recent literary rebels, they merely intended to modify, improve, and renew their disciplines. Although the fellowship reached across many disciplines, and although at first I was the only scientist, in time many scientists joined the fellowship, which continues to be predominantly from literature, music, arts, history, sociology, political science, and law. We were not interdisciplinary; we were multidisciplinary. We did not criticize each other; we criticized ourselves and our fields. There was an appreciation of the other that is rare in a university. Although our fields differed, our way of thinking was shared—to combine a deep commitment to the worthiness of our disciplines with a personal wish to change them. Owen Fiss reflected not on the need for technical changes in the law but on its primary function of creating justice; David Apter spoke of the difficulties of creating democracy in developing countries under the duress of tribal prejudice and residual imperialism; John Boswell spoke of how history could be improved by considering the neglected victims of a time—children in the Middle Ages, like gays and lesbians today, and how by including these outliers history would gain; Paul Frey spoke of the importance of logical thought in poetry, particularly in the Romantic age; and while I listened to the hopes of recreating the values of those disciplines, I struggled with the conflict between what I loved in science and the prevailing assumptions in brain science.

CONSTRUCTIVISM

The outlook at the Humanities Center was to rebuild our disciplines by questioning the assumptions of the several fields represented by the fellowship. Attempts to replace the well-established, unquestioned values were a continuing process

in Western thought, gaining strength in the past century. The classic formulations of knowledge had been in play continuously, emerging and retreating
as new voices appeared in the social sciences, in the humanities, and in science itself. Social studies of science following Thomas Kuhn, Ludwik Fleck,
and Michel Foucault had questioned existing understanding, not as well-struc-
tured, comprehensive new philosophies, but as empirical insights questioning
what had been considered uncontestable. These ideas about science differed
from the Viennese logical positivists and Karl Popper as well as from the earlier
epistemology of Kant and Descartes. This revised conception of understanding,
called constructionism, replaced established views with hypotheses recognized
to be contingent and in need of support.[2] But the act of self-consciously constructing an understanding was being built on the assumptions that there was a
real world out there while our understanding of that world was constructed by
humans in an effort to deal with, understand, and control it. Our understanding, contingent with differing degrees of reliability, was not an effort to recre-
ate something that was to be found in that world, not to mirror it, but was a
human attempt to understand it. The understanding we undertook to find was
not independent of our sensory, perceptual, or conceptual activities but rather,
as Barbara Herrnstein Smith, a leading constructionist, said:

> emerging from...or "constructed by" those activities. In contrast to the
> prevailing assumptions of rationalist philosophy of mind, constructivist
> accounts of cognitive processes see beliefs not as discrete, correct or incor-
> rect propositions about or mental representations of the world but, rather,
> as linked perceptual dispositions and behavioral routines that are con-
> tinuously strengthened, weakened and reconfigured through our ongoing
> interactions with our environments.[2]

She continued that in contrast to considering scientific truths **not** as a match
between "statements or beliefs" and the autonomous features of an external
world, constructivists consider them rather as a "relatively stable and effective mutual coordination among statements, beliefs, experiences and practical
activities." In this view scientific truth and knowledge are not products of an
exclusively privileged method of reasoning but have been constructed with a
high capability of gaining support by testing, experimentation, and understanding. In other words, science shared with other human attempts to understand
the world the construction of hypotheses but had the possibility of particularly
strong interactions with a wide range of observations, beliefs, and effectiveness,
allowing physical science to have a privileged degree of reliability among the
disciplines. In this view a reliable science, like physics or chemistry, has the ability to serve curiosity by constructing explanatory hypotheses that can have a

particularly wide network of support from observation and from their compatibility with wide conceptual networks, each with its own experiential support.

In my first presentation at the Humanities Center, to emphasize the support that scientifically constructed and tested hypotheses can find, I spoke on "The Joy of Error," celebrating science's advantage over literature because our methodology allowed the investigator to disprove a hypothesis; in other words, I appealed to Karl Popper's definition, which he proposed would distinguish science from non-science. They heard me through—and they were very gentle and indulgent, possibly pleased by having a scientist interested, in fact eager, to talk seriously with them. They were kind not to point out how far considerations about disprovability, such as Duhem's, had gone since Popper's early thesis. Duhem had, long before Popper's proposal, shown that the strongly interconnected nature of scientific statements, which as mentioned above was the very source of their strength, interfered with hopes of separating a single feature that could be disproven. But the limitations felt, not by my colleagues but by me, about this simplistic talk, in contrast to the nuanced depths of the humanists' presentations, led me to consider science more carefully than when I started my talk. The continual reevaluation of the goals and styles of serious literary criticism invoked by deconstruction set standards of self-criticism that had consequences for all the disciplines represented by this broad fellowship. I began to sense how epistemological questions were common to both science and the humanities, rendering them more similar than suggested by their subjects. These debates—about how various disciplines determined, discovered, or created something that they considered a "truth"—were not confined to academic disputes and soon merged with administrative decisions. I found myself getting pulled into discussions about campus politics that didn't allow me to remain complaisant about how we scientists did our work.

WESTERN CIVILIZATION AND THE CURRICULUM

In the 1980s Sid Bass, a wealthy Yale alumnus, offered several millions of dollars to support a change in the undergraduate curriculum that would add additional emphasis to Western civilization and would form the basis of a new undergraduate major. This change required Yale faculty approval, and it was discussed and criticized at a lively Yale College faculty meeting. At issue were the profound changes in knowledge and the views of truth that reflected, in the academy, the postcolonial world and the rebellion against authority taking place in the world. The humanistic fields were being enlivened by debates about how the traditional Western cultural canon was showing some cracks. Literary critics were appreciating some aspects of the disruptive questioning of theory, social scientists and anthropologists were appreciating cultures that were once thought of as inferior to the teleological domination of Western empires, social historians were listening to (and appreciating) the voices of women or others who didn't walk the halls of power in the empires. Western civilization was being reinforced by the Bass gift in order to combat what its defenders considered its main threat—the thesis that knowledge is socially constructed and that value judgments were relative and influenced by who held power. The canon of great books had been challenged as part of the increasing belief that our literature, like our values, was constructed by humans and that the curriculum should be modified as the world changed. The gift to strengthen Western civilization directly tried to resist those changes. While the possibility of revising or disregarding the canon of great books was the crucial issue in the academy, and in literature particularly, this issue was symbolic of the challenge to authority that was sweeping society and that had been brought to the streets and campuses by the student uprisings in the sixties. These happenings were still vivid for many of the faculty, and a curriculum change, always controversial, was a polarized topic in this climate.

The Dean of Yale College, in defending the idea of a renewed emphasis on Western civilization, characterized the literature faculty, especially the faction at the Whitney Humanities Center, as antirealists because they believed that truth or values were not to be found but were, in fact, created by humans. One political consequence of social constructivism, feared by its critics, was that the dependence on social origin introduced relativism into values that they considered to contrast with traditional values, assumed to be independent of such variable influences.

In criticizing the humanists for what he described as their relativism, the Dean asserted that, fortunately, standards of truth, not socially conditioned, were still found among scientists, and humanists would be well advised to follow the orderly search for truths that the scientists conducted.

Since my scientific studies had begun to focus on brain/mind issues, I was beginning to understand the limitations of a positivistic scientific methodology. I was beginning to feel that, while scientists have a powerful track record of describing the physical world, we still did not have some mechanical ability to "reveal" a definite truth. We were establishing working truths based on observation and experimentation, but we did so within the boundaries of our field, which gave us the reliability of science but did not give us a privileged position as we moved away from the rewarding everyday practice of our science to the frontiers of scientific understanding, and then beyond to personal and cultural values. Mounting the stage and in a halting voice, I said that I often found that instead of being sure of directions and assumptions because of my scientific training, I often felt uncertainties similar to my friends in the humanities. I did not hold, I said, with the image of scientists sitting at their desks analyzing data and then every so often moving to the salami of truth hanging in their office to cut a slice for publication. The faculty's opposition to the Bass gift was reinforced by similar arguments made that day. The gift was eventually declined and the Dean was soon replaced. I didn't argue in this way because I was against studying the treasures of Western culture (I was not). I didn't assert my views in this way because I doubted that physical science had the capacity to test and validate (by means of observation and consensus) very important and practical working truths (I did not doubt this). I just felt that it was important to assert that the scientific pursuit of truth was an uncertain creative act—and part of that realization was that in the name of that pursuit, one could be unknowingly stuck in some careless assumptions about what we knew.

THE SLIPPERY SLOPE

It was a highly emotional experience, and my dramatic contradiction of the conservative view of science requires some examination. The Dean was express-ing a favorable view of science, in which it held a privileged position when looking for truth. It was, not only for the Dean but for many of my scientist and non-scientist colleagues, quite unexpected for a scientist to throw his lot in with the opponents of the Western canon and to refuse the privileged posi-tion offered to science. In describing science as creating, in fact, constructing its truths, I seemed to dispute the importance of scientific understanding. My hesitancy in disputing the Dean reflected my concern, and that of many of my scientific colleagues, that I was on the slippery slope of relativism, that science was not privileged, but that its beliefs and understandings were constructed by humans, and like all other disciplines was not independent of social forces, while at the same time it was the most reliable method available for under-standing the world.

It took me a while to realize that the slippery slope of constructivism that I instinctively defended was not the enemy of science: it was the ideal of *good* science. In its most original realization, the inductive empirical conduct of sci-ence found understanding by hypothesis testing. At this level scientists were constructivist, with our beliefs depending on conditions where new informa-tion, new data, meant a changed social condition. My dedication to science had been based upon its ability to test hypotheses well enough so as to generate the reliable scientific laws and procedures I had been enthusiastically applying to biology.

My exposure to the similarities of the creative act in science and the humani-ties had been enhanced by 7 years of teaching a course in literature and science with the literary critic Michael Holquist to a mixed class of undergraduate majors in science and the humanities. The varied reading—poems by Wallace Stevens, history by Kuhn and Toulmin, *Fathers and Sons* by Turgenev about the influence of German science of the nineteenth century upon Russia—were all part of the assignments that students wrote about in weekly and term reports. We chose readings from literature with a slant on creativity that did not make comparisons between science and the arts but rather showed their commonalities. It was stimulating to be reading great writers again, with an eye toward what kinds of truth claims they were asserting. Just as I had learned with Trilling (40 years earlier) about the individual defining himself within and against a tradition, within and against a culture, I found the reading of scientists and poets to be saying the same thing. Galileo was supporting the Copernican world against the Church's authority, while 100 years earlier Copernicus had not dared to publish his views. But the piece whose insight for scientific life was most immediate was not Galileo, not *Arrowsmith*, not Huxley, but Oscar Wilde, the favorite reading of the course for students and teacher alike. In his essay "The Decay of Lying," Wilde bemoaned that the quality of lying had slipped, but it was not the everyday lying as practiced by politicians and bad novelists that had shrunk. Rather, he continued, we no longer find the Great Lies in which someone creates something that had never before existed, that contradicts all we had previously believed and becomes recognized because of its meaningfulness for life, as Great Art does. In this felicitous event, Life imitates Art by following the inspired vision. Nothing in our reading could be shown more clearly to illustrate the similarity of the arts and sciences. When Wilde says that "the aim of life is to find self-expression, and that Art offers it certain beautiful forms through which it may realize that energy," we can, by realizing that science offers us the same opportunity, see clearly the similarity between the human usage of science and art.[3] The influence of creative science on life that we see, for example, in the effects of quantum mechanics on our technological world is clearly seen in Wilde's witty essay. This identity of science and art disregarded the muddy differences laid out in Snow's "The Two Cultures" and in the political critiques it spawned. In its place it celebrated the shared simplicity of creating something that had never before existed.

Although there are these fundamental similarities between science and other human creative acts, still at all levels of physical science other than the most unsettled frontier, the Dean was right in crediting science with a unique degree of reliability and certainty. In what Thomas Kuhn characterized as "normal" science, the rules and laws, or paradigms as he called them, are in place. Normal science, in accepting these well-established laws of physical science, has been able to create the technological world and has given us unique certainty. In my analysis of neuroscience I continually emphasize the importance of staying within the boundaries of certainty afforded by chemical and physical experiments and concepts. The great scope of science includes the different degrees of reliability between everyday, normal science and the contingencies at the frontiers of scientific understanding. Nowhere is this range more evident than in neuroscience, whose goal, as explored throughout this book, is to relate subjective processes to the quite objective findings of physical science.

SCIENTISTS AS INTELLECTUALS

Beyond the goals of using philosophy to guide scientific research in the complex interdisciplinary world of modern neuroscience, there is a more personal reason, implicit in my personal history, for an interest in the philosophy animating neuroscience. An awareness of the opposition to culture places the individual in the role of a critic, a position that is less common in science than in other scholarly subjects. In contrast to the continual self-questioning in the social sciences and the humanities as to the value of their discipline, scientists are confident about the value of their field. Scientific life is dominated by criticisms of experimental and theoretical results. But as Thomas Kuhn has emphasized, criticism of the paradigms of a subfield of science is less common than is the continuing evaluation of findings within the field. Criticism of a paradigm like cognitive psychology is uncommon in everyday scientific life. Scientists' criticisms are generally more focused on particular findings.

In contrast to criticism in science, the humanities hold almost continuing conferences on the value of the humanities designed to affirm their value for the world. Classics have been arguing for the importance of teaching Latin for several centuries. Literary criticism has emerged to serve philosophy's traditional role of evaluating the good, the bad, and the beautiful. Its stated objective in many cases has been to show that criticism itself is a worthy subject, whose value is not limited to bringing out the importance of creative literature. Analyses and criticism of science from history, philosophy, and sociology have recently been growing, but there are very few questions raised about the value of "science" by active scientists. A complacency about the unlimited value of science for society and for human civilization in general is not uncommon in the public stance of leading scientists who, when occasionally called on to defend science, answer with unabashed confidence. The usual answer as to what science needs is more money, although occasionally it is supplemented by the need to defend science from creationists and other critics. When the possibility of having discussions about the findings of the field of "science studies" within the annual meetings of the National Academy of Sciences was on the agenda, it was abandoned in response to the pleas of positivistic sociologists who didn't want those camels in their tent. Any reservations about directions being followed by the major scientific culture risk being considered confrontational and siding with its enemies. Open animated discussions about science by scientists from the perspective of the individual in today's world or from the larger vista offered by philosophers past and present are scarce, and individuals harboring those thoughts can be somewhat isolated in the midst of their self-confident colleagues.

The need for neuroscientists to ask questions about the broad directions of their field, to look into the origins, meanings, and usages of the many terms describing mental processes that form the core of neuroscientific enquiry has been emphasized throughout the previous chapters. I propose that science would profit by opening the range of its self-criticism. The influence of previous results on a typical scientific report is shown by the carefully documented references cited in scientific articles and books. But, as shown brilliantly by the great Yale critic of literature, Harold Bloom, the influence of the past is very broad, creating in the great poets and the perceptive scientists questions about what opportunities exist for their contributions in the existing structures created by previous workers. And in the struggle to find their role, in the reflections created by the anxiety about their place, scientists can, and I argue should, follow the larger questions of life and death that the intellectual brings to bear on the immediacies of the moment. In this book I ask practicing scientists to add their personal skills as an intellectual to their armament, to address immediate questions by universal as well as immediate standards. If the person in the street is asked which professionals are intellectuals, scientists will not often be missing from those lists. And of course this judgment is correct—science is the embodiment of reason into life, and scientists strive to follow its laws. But harried contemporary scientists beset by the efforts needed to file grant applications, meet deadlines, promote their work by talks, and listen to others by attending meetings and reading the literature have little energy left to propose and admire the universals that originally drove them to this profession. In my life, welcoming circumstances have fortunately permitted me, in an amateurish but passionate way, to follow the hopes made at an early age in the high school bus.

Galileo's physics remains a precious gift that has been preserved and extended, while his dedication to scientific methods, in the face of opposition, is a renewable, equally valuable resource. In reexamining neuroscientific studies of mental processes I have been supported by his physics and his methods. Suggestions as to how research can further certain goals, such as the interdisciplinary directions supported in this book, must, and will, be judged by their scientific usefulness, not by philosophical judgments. Philosophical insights and similarities with the humanities have been selected for their concordance with and encouragement of the scientific practices advocated. Their value lies in clarifying scientific directions by emphasizing the implications of choosing certain methodologies. But beyond their practical guidance, their meaningfulness for somewhat alienated scientists, rather detached in their judgments about their devoted subject, lies in their reassuring voice, expressing differently and often more clearly the broad values of the science they adore—and therefore criticize.

NOTES

1. Trilling, L. (1965). Beyond culture. In *Freud: Within and beyond culture* (p. 89). New York: Harcourt Brace Jovanovich.
2. Smith, B. H. (2005). *Scandalous knowledge: Science, truth and the human* (Chapter 1). Durham, NC: Duke University Press.
3. Wilde, O. (1994). The decay of lying. In *The complete works of Oscar Wilde* (p. 992). New York: Barnes & Noble.

ACKNOWLEDGMENTS

This book exists because Owen Fiss believed that I had something to say about science, presumably from the shared belief that the personal was the ultimate strength of professionalism. His confidence sustained me for the eight long years it needed. Barbara Herrnstein Smith encouraged my early unformulated but deeply felt writings about brain experiments by her examples of how philosophical understanding could be accurately and logically developed. Her comments on my early drafts moved me closer to having a book. At Oxford University Press, Joan Bossert made helpful suggestions for improving the manuscript and I'm thankful to Miles Osgood for bringing it to publication. Harry Haskell edited some of the early versions of these chapters using his clear intelligence to organize my thinking. Meko Owens-Ward helped in numerous ways by typing, retyping, and finding references. Professors Fahmeed Hyder, Todd Constable, and Douglas Rothman of the Yale Magnetic Resonance Research Center kindly provided the figures used for the cover.

My advocacy of certain scientific directions, and criticism of others, came from a long scientific career during which a talented group of collaborators developed noninvasive fMRI and MRS imaging of the brain. Since he came as a graduate student to Yale thirty years ago, attracted to the possible future of these studies, Doug Rothman has been a continuing companion, building ideas and experiments, actually developing the equipment, and getting the experiments done. He created and directed the Yale Magnetic Resonance Research Center where the experiments have been done that made this book possible. Fahmeed Hyder and Kevin Behar have been the primary sources of strength and knowledge among the many at Yale who contributed to the brain studies reviewed in this book. Other significant scientific contributions to the development of Magnetic Resonance Spectroscopy and fMRI at Yale have been made by Nicola Sibson, Graeme Mason, Wei Chen, Rolf Gruetter, Andrew Blamire, Susan Fitzpatrick, Ognen Petroff, James Pritchard, Edward Novotny, Gregory McCarthy, Patricia Goldman-Rakic, Fuqiang Xu, Ikuhiro Kida, Hoby Hetherington, Hadassah Degani, Anant Patel, Bruce Wexler, Elizabeth Phelps, Xiao-Hong Zhu, Yiaojin Yang, Ajay Dhankhar, James Schafer, Pieter van Eijdsen, Christoph Juchem, Robin deGraaf, Natasha Maandag, Hal Blumenfeld, Jun Shen, Takashi Ogino, Thomas Jue, Youngran Chun, Malcolm J. Avison, Norman Siegal, Michael

Stromski, Jullie Pan, Maren Laughlin, Jacqueline K Barton, Jeff Alger, Li-Hsin Zhang, Thomas Price, Yair Shachar-Hill, and Jan Den Hollander.

The brain metabolic studies by fMRI and Magnetic Resonance Spectroscopy were a continuation of earlier research at Bell Laboratories on simpler systems. There, several brilliant and courageous young scientists chose to develop the promise offered by the rudimentary area of *in vivo* metabolism in more accessible systems like bacteria, yeast, and perfused organs. I am particularly appreciative of the collaborations with Gil Navon, Seiji Ogawa, Kamil Ugurbil, Tetsue Yamane, Kurt Wuthrich, Joseph Eisinger, Truman Brown, Sheila M. Cohen, Robert J. Gillies, Jim Salhany, and Kees Hilbers.

At Bell Laboratories I enjoyed the excitement of science with Phil Anderson and a long collaboration with John Hopfield that set standards for scientific creativity during those days and in memory since. I moved away from condensed matter physics, with help from the John Simon Guggenheim Foundation, to apply well-established laws of thermodynamics and quantum mechanics to the mechanisms of biological phenomena. As a result of studying mechanisms, this book is about partial causes and incomplete explanations, which I consider suitable for the scientific state of our subject. I was encouraged in the hope that understanding this book did not need a thorough understanding of science but required only intelligence, imagination, and curiosity when my son James L. Shulman, who evidences these rare qualities, turned out to be my most valuable reader and adviser. James carefully edited all the chapters and ensured that, at least in its own terms, the book made sense. I thank my son Mark R. Shulman for clarifying several of my ideas. I very much appreciated comments from Professor Maxwell R. Bennett on several crucial points.

My wife, Stephanie Spangler, supported me by her confidence in the value of this endeavor and by her understanding of the effort and was always encouraging, loving, and helpful. I am continually aware of my good fortune in being in the United States of America during these years and of enjoying the support for long-term research goals offered by the Bell Telephone Laboratories and Yale University.

Robert G. Shulman
January 1, 2013